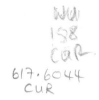

Handbook of
Dental Trauma
A practical guide to the tre͟   ͟ ͟ͅrauma to the teeth

Handbook of
Dental Trauma
A practical guide to
the treatment of trauma to the teeth

Edited by   M.E.J. Curzon

Authors: M.E.J. Curzon BDS MSc PhD FRCD(C) FDSRCS
M.S. Duggal BDS MDS PhD FDS(Paeds) RCS
S.A. Fayle BDS MDSc MRCD(C) FDSRCS
K.J. Toumba BSc BChD MSc PhD FDSRCS

with   E. A. O'Sullivan BChD MDentSci PhD MRCD(C)
contributions by FDS(Paeds) RCS
J.F. Tahmassebi BDS MDSc FRCD(C)
Department of Paediatric Dentistry,
Leeds Dental Institute,
University of Leeds.

wright

OXFORD AUCKLAND BOSTON JOHANNESBURG MELBOURNE NEW DELHI

Wright
An imprint of Butterworth-Heinemann
Linacre House, Jordan Hill, Oxford OX2 8DP
225 Wildwood Avenue, Woburn, MA 01801-2041
A division of Reed Educational and Professional Publishing Ltd

ℛ A member of the Reed Elsevier plc group

First published 1999

British Library Cataloguing in Publication Data
A catalogue record for this book is available from the British Library

Library of Congress Cataloguing in Publication Data
A catalogue record for this book is available from the Library of Congress

ISBN 0 7236 1741 4

Typeset by Keytec Typesetting Ltd, Bridport, Dorset
Printed and bound in Great Britain by MPG Books Ltd, Bodmin, Cornwall

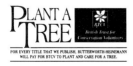

PLANT A TREE

British Trust for
Conservation Volunteers

FOR EVERY TITLE THAT WE PUBLISH, BUTTERWORTH-HEINEMANN
WILL PAY FOR BTCV TO PLANT AND CARE FOR A TREE.

Contents

Preface

Over the years we have taught a number of courses or given lectures to dental practitioners and to undergraduate and postgraduate students on dental trauma. From this experience we have compiled this practical guide for the efficient and successful handling of children, and older patients, with trauma. Our intention is to provide a protocol that dentists in practice can use to ensure that any patient who presents with damaged teeth will receive the best possible care, but at the same time without seriously disrupting the smooth running of the dentist's practice.

Trauma to the teeth in children and adolescents poses a problem to many general dental practitioners and community dental officers. By the very nature of the circumstances surrounding such injuries, they are completely unplanned. The child or adolescent arrives at the dentist's practice distressed, perhaps in shock, and needing immediate attention. Yet the dentist is inevitably already busy with a full appointment book. At the same time, while we see patients with broken teeth virtually every day, for the dental practitioner this is not a frequent occurrence. Accordingly the treatment of broken teeth is not a skill that the practitioner can improve by frequent practice. There is therefore a need for a structured response that ensures the efficient handling of these dental trauma cases.

The approach is to provide a handbook and not an extensive scientifically based textbook. Therefore, in this handbook we provide simple instructions that we hope can be read quickly and also that can be used at the chairside to aid in the care of a patient with fractured teeth. We acknowledge that we have not delved into the scientific background and rationale for each procedure. This is dealt with very effectively in the much larger textbooks on traumatic injuries already available for those students wishing to study the subject in depth. Rather, we have taken the approach that busy practitioners, and undergraduate and postgraduate students, need a ready reference guide that can be kept close at hand. This will help them provide the standard of care needed on those infrequent occasions when a patient arrives in their practice with damaged teeth.

MEJC, MSD, SAF, KJT

Acknowledgements

Much of the illustrative material for this handbook has been derived from clinical material carried out by staff and students of the department of Paediatric Dentistry at Leeds. These illustrations were largely taken by the staff of the Leeds Dental Hospital, Audio-Visual Department, of our patients, under the direction of Angus Robertson. His contribution and that of his staff is very gratefully acknowledged. No matter what the request for photographs was, the Audio-Visual Department has always been able to willingly help. The drawings were expertly done by Anna Durban of the same department. We are also indebted to Dr Jane Wynn, Paediatrician of the Leeds General Infirmary, and Dr Muir Martin for contributing photographs concerned with non-accidental injuries.

We are very appreciative of the support of our clinical staff and students and their help in the preparation of this book. A number of other people have also helped us with its preparation. In particular we would wish to thank Dr John Tiernan of *Dental Protection* for valuable advice and suggestions on the chapter dealing with the legal implications of trauma.

Chapter 1

Introduction: history taking, diagnosis and treatment planning

M.E.J. Curzon

The typical case of trauma to the anterior teeth appears at the dentist's office or surgery late in a morning, or afternoon, when the schedule of patients is already running late for the day. The staff are very busy with booked-in patients and yet here is an emergency to be cared for. A confounding issue in these trauma cases is that for the great majority of general dental practitioners dental trauma is a relatively rare event. Dental practices specializing in paediatric dentistry are well versed in the care of these patients, but a general dental practice, experiencing less than perhaps one a month, has the problem of keeping staff up to scratch with the necessary techniques. Each case of dental trauma is different from the one seen previously: some are complex and some are simple. It is unlikely that any typical general dental practice will see enough cases to become adept at treating them without some formalized programme to provide the standards of care needed.

This textbook seeks to aid the busy dentist by providing a simple guide to treating broken and damaged teeth and soft tissues. This can be accomplished by laying out simple protocols and guidelines for a step-by-step approach to the efficient care of traumatized teeth.

THE TYPICAL SITUATION

The child, teenager or young adult arriving at the door of the dental practice may be in a state of shock, with facial tissues that are grazed or lacerated and with damaged teeth. A parent or friend is with them, who is often more anxious and upset than the patient, and demands that something be done *immediately*.

The dentist is presented with the problem of dealing with this emergency as quickly and efficiently as possible and yet at the same time continuing to look after the other patients already being seen. This scenario can be dealt with in one of three ways:

- the patient is refused treatment and told to find another dentist;
- the patient is referred to another dentist or specialist clinic where the necessary treatment can be carried out;
- the patient is treated promptly and efficiently in the practice which then generates further goodwill for the dentist concerned.

The disadvantage of the first two scenarios is that the patient's treatment is delayed, which may seriously compromise the chances of successful treatment. The sooner many fractures of the teeth are treated, the greater the chance of success (Hamilton *et al.*, 1997). In addition, the perception will be generated by the patient, parents or friends that the dentist is not receptive to caring for patients in an emergency. This is in contrast to the third scenario, where the patient is quickly and efficiently cared for, with a successful outcome. Research has shown that if trauma involves the pulp of a tooth and treatment is initiated quickly the success rate is over 60%, but reduces to only 10% if treatment is delayed (Oulis and Berdouses, 1996).

Yet, as noted above, patients with orofacial trauma seldom attend a dentist at the most convenient time. Therefore, those dentists who are caring and able to treat children and adults with damaged or fractured teeth are successfully well prepared. They have planned beforehand so that they and their staff know exactly what to do in the most efficient way that requires the least disruption of the normal workings of the practice, but provides high-quality care for damaged or fractured teeth.

PROTOCOLS

Just as a dental practice these days must have protocols, or standard operating procedures (SOPs), for the management of cross-infection control, storage and keeping of drugs, sterilizing procedures, etc., so a well-organized practice should have a **trauma protocol** for the management of orofacial trauma. Such a document should be drawn up by the dental team and reviewed at periodic intervals so that each member knows exactly what is their role. Each new member of staff should be required to study all the SOPs of the practice, and a periodic review should be conducted to keep all staff up to date. In the case of orofacial trauma, these events require all members of the team, from receptionist to dentist, to function in a prescribed way so that the dental treatment is carried out efficiently and all the necessary documentation is completed to a high standard, but at the same time without delaying the care of the traumatized patient or other patients.

Remember, patients with a trauma injury will be upset, distressed and may be in shock.

Empathy and a caring attitude are essential.

1 **Receptionist**. Welcome patient and accompanying persons; seat in waiting room; determine immediate problem:
   What sort of injury – teeth, lips, gums, face?
   Teeth involved – when, where, what time today?
   Tell dentist that case of trauma has arrived
   Obtain trauma form and set of dental records (or old dental records if already a patient). Fill out Part 1 of the trauma form.
   Reassure patient that they will be seen as soon as possible.
2 **Dental nurse**. When notified that a trauma patient has arrived, check on type of trauma. Fill out Part 2 of trauma form.
   Prepare: examination kit, vitality testing – electronic, ethyl chloride, local analgesia, rubber dam splinting materials/kit.
   Tell dentist when all is ready.
   Bring patient into surgery, get them seated and comfortable.
   Assist dentist in completion of trauma form and examination.
3 **Dentist**. Completion of assessment, trauma form and initial diagnosis.
   Decision is made to:
   (A) **Treat today** – needs radiograph, local analgesia, restoration, pulp treatment, splinting.
   (B) **Emergency treatment today only** – dress tooth/teeth, reappoint in ? days.
   (C) **No immediate treatment now** – reappoint in ? days.
   Completion of trauma form – make sure *all* sections are completed, form is signed, radiographs are filed with trauma form, follow-up appointment(s) have been made.
4 **Follow-up**. There must be follow-up appointments; time periods for these are:
   (A) uncomplicated crown fracture (enamel or enamel/dentine) to be seen in 1 month.
   (B) complicated crown fracture, no displacement injury to be seen in 1 month.
   (C) displacement injury with or without splint, root fracture with splint to be seen in 1 week.
   (D) tissue lacerations with sutures to be seen in 1 week.
5 **Splinting**. Splints must be retained for an appropriate period of time:
   (A) displacement injuries with physiological splint, retain for 1 week.
   (B) root fractures, splint for 8 weeks.
   (C) avulsion plus apical root fracture, splint for 10 days.

Figure 1.1 An example of a trauma protocol

A sample protocol is shown in Figure 1.1. This should not be regarded as a prescribed design of protocol, but is only given here as an example that may be modified for local circumstances. The protocol should be typed and kept in the SOP manual within the main reception area of the dental practice.

It is useful to have a dry run, or practice, of the treatment of these patients. In an efficient practice these rehearsals should occur anyway for all the SOPs used. The care of dental trauma is to some extent in a special category because these cases are emergencies that require **rapid treatment** in order to ensure maximum success. Practice makes perfect in all aspects of dental care.

ROLES OF THE DENTAL TEAM

Receptionist

This person is the first to see the patient presenting with facial trauma. The receptionist should immediately welcome the patient to the dental practice and sit him/her comfortably in the waiting area. Sympathy should be expressed over this sudden and unexpected event and a promise of immediate treatment made. The receptionist should then identify the exact date, time and place of the injury. If it occurred several days before, then the urgency for immediate treatment is much less. Trauma that occurred that very day, and within the previous three hours, means that more immediate care is called for.

Once having settled the patient and parent/friend, the receptionist notifies the dentist that a trauma case has arrived and, if possible, the outline nature of the injury. This may be simply:

- a broken tooth;
- damaged face and gums;
- a tooth knocked out;
- a considerable amount of damage to face and teeth.

The clinical dental staff do not need to stop immediately what they are doing, as this is detrimental to the patient(s) already under their care. However, a brief conversation between dentist(s) and dental nurse(s) should establish how quickly the treatment of the patient already in the surgery and being treated can be completed, or halted for a few minutes while the care of the traumatized patient is started.

It is at this juncture that the use of a **trauma form** (Figure 1.2) proves to be essential for the efficient practice. In assessing a case of dental trauma, it is unfortunately necessary to bear in mind that there may well be legal implications that will occur months, or even years, after the event (see Chapter 3). While accurate dental records are mandatory in any dental practice, for the care of dental trauma they are absolutely imperative. This importance cannot be more highly stressed. However, the completion of paperwork takes time and here

TRAUMA HISTORY AND DIAGNOSIS FORM

Part I   Receptionist

Name ....Today's Date ..../..../....

Referral Source...

History of Injury

Date of injury ..../..../....   Time ....

Location..

Cause..

Part II   Dental Nurse

Nature of Dental Injury..

Other Injuries? .... KO'd? Yes/No

Previous dental opinion/treatment? ....

....

Radiographs?.....................Drugs ? ....

Symptoms now?...

Nausea/dizziness/diplopia?................................

HISTORY- dental ....

         medical ....

Part III   Dentist

EXAMINATION

Extra-oral

    Soft tissues ....

    Facial Skeleton ....

    Mandibular.movement/occlusion ....

Intra-oral

    Soft tissues ....

    Oral hygiene/perio status ....

Teeth Present (full charting)

	8	7	6	5	4	3	2	1	1	2	3	4	5	6	7	8	
	8	7	6	5	4	3	2	1	1	2	3	4	5	6	7	8	
	8	7	6	5	4	3	2	1	1	2	3	4	5	6	7	8	

Injuries to teeth ....

....

Injuries to soft tissues ....

....

Figure 1.2 (see also overleaf)

the role of the receptionist becomes essential. A well-designed trauma form is laid out in such a way that a dental auxiliary can record much of the necessary information before the dentist needs to see the patient.

Once the preliminary paperwork has been completed by the receptionist, the patient can be admitted to the dental office/surgery. The time taken to complete the trauma form has allowed the dental nurse(s) to prepare a dental chair for the new patient or to finish the

Part IV   Trauma Form Page 2
Teeth Injured

Tooth	Clinical Injury	Vitality Tests Eth.Cl ETP	Mobility	TTP	Transill-umination	Root dev stage *

Vitality	Mobility	TTP	Tranaillumination	Root Dev Stage
- = no	Grade 0-3	0 = nil	N = normal	1 = $<^2/_3$
N = normal		+ = yes		2 = $>^2/_3$
+ = hypersens		+ + = severe		3 = complete (apex open)
			ANK = ankylosis	4 = complete (apex closed)

Avulsion Only
Extra alveolar Period ....
Method of storage...

Radiographs   Views: OPT. . . . .   PA. . . . . .   Soft Tiss. . . . . . .
Report...
....
....
....

Diagnosis

Tooth	Diagnosis

Treatment Plan
....
....
....
....
....
....

SIGNED   . . . . .Date . ./. ./ . .

Figure 1.2 *continued*

care of an existing patient with an appointment. Obviously a dental practice with several chairs has an advantage in these circumstances.

Dental nurse

Having been advised by the receptionist that there is a trauma case to be accommodated into the patient schedule, the nurse now needs to

Part V
FOLLOW-UP TREATMENT

Trauma Form Page 3

Name ....

Time after injury (*Enter date*)	Xrays	Vitality tests Eth. Chl ETP		Mobility	Transill/ colour	TTP	Photos
1 wk							
3 wks	*						
6 wks							
3 mths	*						
6 mths							
1 yr	*						
2 yrs							
3 yrs							

Further follow-up visits would usually occur at 5,10 and 15 yrs

* indicates minimum radiographic requirement

LEGAL REPORTS

Solicitor	Typed	Date Sent
1.........................		
2.........................		
3.........................		
4.........................		
5.........................		

Figure 1.2 *continued*

prepare for this treatment. In most cases radiographs, usually periapical views, will need to be taken. Sensibility (vitality) tests with ethyl chloride, or electronic testing, may be required (Chapter 2). There may well be a need for local analgesia. A rubber dam will be imperative if there is pulpal involvement of any fractured teeth. In cases of displacement, luxation or avulsion injuries a splint will need

Part VI   Trauma Form Page 4

NAI RECORDS   Completed by . . . .

Name . . . .   **Date** . . ./. . ./. . .

Parent/Guardian/Carer(s) Present . . . .

. . . .

History of Accident as Given by Parent/Carer

. . . .

. . . .

. . . .

. . . .

. . . .

. . . .

Witness(s) to injuries . . . .

Observations on Manner and Dress of Child

. . . .

. . . .

. . . .

. . . .

Summary of Dental Injuries

. . . .

. . . .

Signs of Other Injuries

. . . .

. . . .

Report of Injuries given to:

1. . . . . .telephone . . . . in writing . . . . . .

2. . . . . .telephone . . . . in writing . . . . . .

3. . . . . .telephone . . . . in writing . . . . . .

Record of Follow-Up

. . . .

. . . .

Figure 1.2 *continued*

to be placed. All of these require the preparation of the necessary instruments, medicaments and equipment.

Accordingly the dental nurse's role is to ensure that when the patient is brought into the surgery, whatever the dentist will need is ready.

Dental practices that treat considerable numbers of trauma cases may well find that it is convenient to have a trauma kit always available. Indeed where there may be an after-hours service for such patients, sometimes requiring attendance at accident and emergency departments of local hospitals, a portable kit can be made up and kept on hand for the dentist to carry (see Figure 11.8).

Having prepared all the possible immediate requirements for instruments, etc., the dental nurse brings in the patient, seats them and continues to complete the next sections of the trauma form preparatory to the arrival of the dentist. This will also mean the completion of the practice's **medical history form**. In many cases of dental trauma the patient is often new to the practice. Therefore it is essential that a comprehensive medical history is taken.

An important question to ask, as part of the medical history of a trauma case, is whether the tetanus immunization is up to date. In most cases of dental trauma the accident occurred out of doors, perhaps on a playing field, and therefore soil contamination of facial wounds may have occurred. The tetanus vaccination should therefore be up to date. If not, the dental nurse must notify the dentist and arrangements made for a booster as soon as possible.

The dentist

As the preliminary parts of the history and trauma form have already been completed, the dentist is able to complete the more specialized parts of the diagnosis. Again the use of the trauma form aids the memory. This history needs to be taken as quickly and efficiently as possible so that the treatment, if needed, can be started to gain the best prognosis. This will be particularly important in cases of avulsion or severe displacements.

The dentist completes the initial dental examination which serves to identify quickly into which category of dental trauma the patient falls. A suggested list, but not exhaustive is:

- Primary dentition only, child under the age of 5 years:
  - simple fracture of enamel only or enamel–dentine;
  - displacement injury of primary tooth.
- Permanent/mixed dentition, permanent teeth only involved:
  - simple fracture, enamel–dentine only;
  - complicated crown fracture, no displacement of the teeth;
  - displacement/avulsion of one or more permanent teeth.
- Multiple injuries involving teeth and soft tissues.

Depending on this initial diagnosis, the dentist must quickly decide whether active treatment is needed now to enhance the chances of a successful outcome, or whether the patient can wait for a while longer before any treatment is started. For example, a simple small enamel–dentine crown fracture that does not need immediate repair may wait. Periapical radiographs, in this type of case, will show whether there are any root fractures, but a simple small enamel–dentine chip could be put off to a booked appointment within the next few days.

Displacement injuries which need repositioning, such as luxations or avulsions, need immediate attention (assuming that the tooth was knocked out or displaced within the previous two hours). If immediate treatment for an avulsion is not possible, the dentist must ask for the tooth (teeth) to be placed into a suitable medium (milk, saline) until he or she can reimplant the tooth (see Chapter 7). With a written office protocol, the dental staff will know exactly what to do.

The next step, once the dentist has made the decision for immediate or later treatment, is for the dental staff to continue the management of the case. This means the dental nurse can gently clean up the facial tissues, if necessary, getting the patient comfortably seated, preparing local analgesia, radiographs to be taken by the dentist, or taking them herself where legally empowered, and all the time constantly reassuring the patient and accompanying parent or friend that all will be quickly and speedily resolved.

STAGING OF DENTAL TREATMENT

It may be best to stage the dental treatment over the next hour or so. This means that perhaps local analgesia can be given to start the process of analgesia and the dentist then leaves the chairside to see another patient (provided that the other patient does not require a prolonged and difficult procedure), or a radiograph may be taken and the patient left quietly seated while it is processed. Perhaps the initial preparation for the repair of an enamel–dentine fracture can be started and a dentine protective agent applied and the final restoration left for later while a further booked patient is seen.

In the treatment of dental trauma it is more efficient to have any immediate care provided very quickly and then the patient left, but observed, while other patients for regular dental work are seen. This does not upset the trauma patient but rather the measured, steady but sequenced work reassures the patient that all is under control. At the same time the regularly booked patient does not feel that they are being neglected or pushed aside, however sympathetic they may be to the plight of the trauma patient. The reverse where, in a semi-panic, temporary treatment is rushed, serves no good purpose. The work carried out will be second rate, will probably fail and the trauma patient loses a tooth or teeth that might otherwise have been kept. The dentist becomes tense because he or she is getting behind with their other work and the trauma patient feels that insufficient attention has been paid to their very real needs affecting their front teeth with all the aesthetic connotations that will go with saving or losing a front tooth.

The measured use of a trauma protocol and trauma form ensure that the best treatment possible is provided.

RECORD KEEPING

It has already been emphasized that good records are needed. This may seem an unecessarily detailed approach, but will be essential if litigation occurs (see Chapter 3). Specific details to be recorded include:

- who was present at the accident;
- location;
- time of day and who else, or what agent (vehicle, object, etc.), was responsible;
- storage medium, whether any teeth were placed in a storage medium and for how long, and was the storage immediate or later?

The time lapsed between injury and treatment is of paramount importance to ultimate success, as has been well documented by Andreasen and Andreasen (1994). All the past research studies have shown that when traumatized teeth are treated as quickly as possible, the prognosis is improved. It is for these reasons that any delay between accident and initial treatment should be recorded.

It is very important that all sections of the trauma form be completed. This may seem to be unnecessary sometimes and a dentist may be tempted, because of time constraints, to only briefly record the minimum detail when the trauma has been slight, perhaps only a minor infraction or enamel chip. However, it is often these very cases of apparently minor injury where death of the pulp tissue occurs at a later date and the dentist finds that he or she has totally inadequate initial contact records. It is such cases that perhaps some three to five years later may require a detailed legal report.

Medical history

A medical history should be taken as soon as possible. The dental staff need to determine if there are any medical conditions that might complicate the treatment of the trauma. Conditions which might be important are bleeding disorders, heart disease, auto-immune or immunosuppression conditions.

Loss of consciousness

If loss of consciousness has occurred it is important to record whether it was at the time of the injury or later. Concussion can occur quite some time after a head injury. If the patient continues to show signs of drowsiness, a medical opinion or further investigation is required as soon as possible. Under these circumstances the immediate treatment of the dental injury would be simply to stabilize the dental condition. Emergency splinting of displaced or reimplanted avulsed teeth can be achieved very quickly using a splint with Pro-Temp II (see Chapter 11).

Previous treatment

Another aspect of the trauma history should include details as to any previous treatment that has already been completed and by whom. The knowledge of emergency treatment of damaged teeth is increasing among the general population. In many instances school nurses, teaching staff or nurses in accident and emergency departments of hospitals all have some idea of what immediate treatment is called for. It has therefore become increasingly common for some form of initial care to have been carried out. This should be recorded.

Previous attempts, successful or otherwise, to reimplant avulsed teeth, and by whom, should be recorded. Alternatively if the tooth or teeth have been placed in a storage medium for transportation this also needs recording and a note of the length of time in the medium. Current research shows that whether a tooth is kept dry or wet and the length of time before reimplantation determine the prognosis of the treatment (see Chapter 7).

Prescribed drugs

Where any drugs have been prescribed related to, or affecting, the injury this needs to be noted. There are cases where the facial injury may have been seen first by a general medical practitioner who will often prescribe an antibiotic and analgesic prior to referring the patient to a dentist for treatment.

Cause of the injury

The causes of dental injuries are many and varied. Data from the literature shows that most dental injuries are related to sports, play and related activities in children and adolescents (Andreasen and Andreasen, 1994). A note should be made of the cause of the accident as reported by the victim, and if another individual was involved this should also be noted. The names of all other parties, if known, should be recorded. In most cases this information can be obtained by suitably trained receptionists and dental nurses.

In small children of pre-school age, non-accidental injury (NAI) should be considered. This topic is dealt with in detail in Chapter 14. However, NAI can also occur in older children and this should also be borne in mind, although for the general dental practitioner this is likely to be a very rare event.

BEHAVIOUR MANAGEMENT OF TRAUMA CASES

When a child or adolescent attends a dental practice with traumatized teeth or facial tissues they are sometimes upset, in pain and may be in shock. The behavioural management aspects of treatment are there-fore very important. As noted earlier, it is essential to take into consideration how the patient is to be treated but at the same time how to manage the distress. Many children will not have experienced any prior dental treatment, other than check-ups, and this will include local analgesia.

It may well be that a child is unmanageable and cannot be treated. These cases are rare and will need to be referred as quickly as possible to the nearest hospital with a dental department. It is more likely that the child will be quite passive and wanting something to be done as soon as possible. In other cases it may only need a period of settling down, with an explanation as to what is to happen, for the child to be willing to accept treatment.

In virtually all cases of complex or displacement injuries (see Chapters 5–10), local analgesia will be required. With the exception of infractions and small chips of enamel, a traumatized tooth will be sensitive to any operative procedures. All treatment involving the pulp, displacements that require repositioning and avulsions will need profound local analgesia. This should be accomplished by using a topical ointment of benzocaine followed by infiltration of an anaesthetic solution. Lignocaine would be the preferred local anaes-thetic agent as it provides a long-lasting effect. As noted earlier in this chapter, the treatment of traumatized teeth always needs to be fitted into the existing appointment schedule in a general dental practice. Therefore a long-lasting anaesthetic should be used. This allows the dentist to leave the patient while the local analgesia takes effect so that he or she can see another patient until the tooth and tissues are numb.

Local analgesia technique

The technique that is required is simply a maxillary or mandibular infiltration using standard procedures (Fayle and Pollard, 1995). The use of a topical anaesthetic cream, preferably a flavoured one, is highly recommended. As with all aspects of child management in dentistry, painless local analgesia is essential. In the case of trauma to the teeth, the patient's cooperation is absolutely necessary in order to carry out the repair procedures as efficiently and thoroughly as possible.

In the maxilla it is advisable also to infiltrate local anaesthetic solution for the incisive papilla. In the younger child this should be carried out separately. The first stage of an infiltration is performed in the buccal sulcus in the normal way. After a few minutes a further injection is carried out by injecting through the interdental papillae but over the crest of the alveolar bone and through into the region of the incisive papilla. It is not advisable to inject directly into the incisal foramen in young patients as this can be quite painful.

In teenage patients and young adults the need for behaviour management is less. They are usually well able to tolerate the necessary treatment to restore their broken teeth. They are conscious of the need for the cosmetic appearance of a nice set of front teeth and will cooperate accordingly. However, there is unfortunately an in-between group of pre-teens (10–13 years of age) who are dental phobics for whatever reason. Even though their teeth have been badly damaged, they are quite unable to cooperate. In these cases the patient will need to be referred on as quickly as possible to a dental department of a hospital for the treatment to be carried out under general anaesthesia.

Procedure for local analgesia

The step-by-step procedure is as follows:

- Use a '**tell, show, do**' technique to explain what will be done.
- Tell the child the **reasons** why you need to 'put the tooth to sleep' or to 'numb it' if the child is older.

- Place **topical benzocaine** anaesthetic cream; let the child choose the flavour.
- Wait for about 1 minute, or as needed, talking to the child all the time, **explaining** what is going to be done in words appropriate to the child's age.
- Give the **injection of local anaesthetic** agent.
- Leave the child with parent and/or dental nurse and see another patient, approximately 20–30 minutes.
- Return and check that there is **profound anaesthesia**.
- **Repeat or add** local anaesthetic solution if needed.
- Take **radiograph(s)** as indicated.

Another patient should be seen, if possible, while the radiograph(s) is being processed, about 10–15 minutes. Then the anaesthesia should be checked before commencing repairs of damaged tooth/teeth.

Sedation

Sometimes a child, or even an older patient, is very upset and may be crying and uncooperative. There are many reasons for apprehension, such as a strange environment, fear of the unknown, or previous poor experiences when attending a dentist, although it may well be that this is the first time that a child has seen a dentist. In these cases it may be necessary to spend a few minutes calming the child down using normal behavioural techniques (Wright *et al.*, 1987). These should include: 'tell, show, do' (TSD), positive reinforcement, desensitization, etc.

Inhalation sedation (relative analgesia)

A few children cannot be calmed by these methods and, because early treatment is often essential, alternative behavioural techniques may be needed. These may include some form of sedation (Melamed and Quinn, 1994). In many dental practices, relative analgesia (RA) is available and can be used for these children. A short introduction to the use of RA is required and then the child/adolescent is left for a few minutes, under the observation of a dental nurse, to get used to the RA.

A disadvantage of using RA, however, is that there has to be a nose mask to maintain the flow of gases and this may interfere with the upper lip retraction which might be needed during repair of the teeth. The only way to handle this problem is to achieve a sufficient depth of sedation with RA and then to move the nose mask away intermittently so as to carry out treatment.

In some patients RA may only be needed for the period of time when an injection is to be given. Once an adequate depth of analgesia has been obtained the RA apparatus can be switched off, after two minutes of oxygen administration, and the nose mask removed. Where a child has presented with an avulsed tooth, RA may be usefully administered up until the time of tooth reimplantation and then stopped when the splinting is to be carried out. Most cases of dental trauma involve the maxillary incisors and splinting will require retraction of the upper lip for access and the RA mask may get in the way of this. Again, the nose mask may need to be moved intermittently to accommodate this procedure.

In yet other trauma cases, when suturing injuries to the lips, usually the lower lip, sedation is needed and the use of RA is very useful in helping a distressed patient cope with the sensations and discomfort involved in the closing of a wound. Similarly the treatment of cuts, lacerations or severe grazes to the face is benefited by the use of RA during the most painful aspects.

Where RA is not available in a dental practice either alternative approaches have to be used, such as oral sedation (see below), or the patient will have to be referred to another dental practice where such facilities are available or to the nearest hospital containing a dental unit that can provide specialist services. In the last two cases this will be, ideally, a consultant paediatric dentist or an oral surgeon. However, even in these cases some form of emergency treatment is needed to enhance the prognosis.

Oral sedation

An alternative to RA is the use of oral sedation. There are a number of drugs available but their disadvantages, in trauma cases, are that they usually take up to an hour to work and have about a 70% level of effectiveness. Currently the drug of choice would be midazolam, but many other drugs are available (Melamed and Quinn, 1994). Sedative drugs are best used where the stomach is empty or when it is at least two to three hours since food was last ingested. In patients attending with traumatized teeth, this may or may not be the case. The time delay in waiting for an oral sedative to take effect may jeopardize the prognosis of the treatment to be provided. In the experience of the authors, oral sedation is only indicated for minor dental trauma where a delay of over an hour will not materially affect the treatment indicated.

SUMMARY

The treatment of dental trauma requires a rapid assessment of the case and treatment required. The use of a rehearsed trauma protocol is essential so that all members of the dental team know their role and function. Records should be accurate and detailed and the use of a trauma form is highly recommended. With good planning the treatment of dental trauma can be staged so as to accommodate the ongoing dental care of other patients in the dental practice.

REFERENCES

Andreasen, J.O. and Andreasen, F.M. (1994) *Textbook and Colour Atlas of Traumatic Injuries to the Teeth*, 3rd edn. Munksgaard, Copenhagen

Fayle, S.A. and Pollard, M.A. (1995) Local analgesia. In *Restorative Techniques in Paediatric Dentistry*. Martin Dunitz, London

Hamilton, F.A., Hill, F.J. and Holloway, P.J. (1997) An investigation of dento-trauma and its treatment in an adolescent population. Parts 1 and 2. *British Dental Journal*, **182**, 91–95, 129–133

Melamed, S.F. and Quinn, C.L. (1994) *Sedation. A Guide to Patient Management*, 3rd edn. Mosby, St Louis

Oulis, C.J. and Berdouses, E.D. (1996) Dental injuries of permanent teeth treated in private practice in Athens. *Endodontics and Dental Traumatology*, **12**, 60–65

Wright, G.Z., Starkey, P.E. and Gardener, D.E. (1987) *Child Management in Dentistry*, Dental Practition Handbook Series. Wright, Bristol

Chapter 2
Special tests: radiographs and sensibility (vitality) testing

M.E.J. Curzon

In virtually all patients presenting with trauma involving the teeth, as well as soft tissue injuries in many cases, there will be a need for radiographs. In our experience this is an aspect of dental treatment where general dental practitioners do not take enough radiographs. The explanation for this is based on the comments made at the beginning of Chapter 1, in that dentists are usually very busy when a trauma case presents in their dental practice. There is a great temptation not to bother with taking any radiographs. Unfortunately many injuries involving exposures of the pulp, root fractures or damage to the alveolar bone are therefore missed. On subsequent visits, pathological changes to the roots and nerve canals can be left undiagnosed. Furthermore, radiographs are extremely important to monitor continued root growth in young permanent incisors. A continuation of root development, after trauma, signifies a vital pulp, irrespective of the results of sensibility (vitality) tests.

A similar situation occurs with sensibility tests. It may often be necessary to check the vitality of the teeth periodically over many weeks or months, but this is usually not done. Evidence of pulp healing may be gained from repeated sensibility tests taken over several months. Once again, however, general dental practitioners are often neglectful of this simple test.

FREQUENCY OF RADIOGRAPHS AND SENSIBILITY TESTS

Obviously radiographs are needed at the time of the first visit with the presentation of the trauma. It is a great mistake not to take any radiographs at this first visit, even though the presenting symptom may be only a tiny chip of enamel or an infraction (see Chapter 4). It is very simple injuries that become neglected, not followed up and the pulpal tissues left to die slowly. In due course the patient returns with a periapical abscess of apparently unknown origin. Unless the soft tissue injuries are considerable or the child/patient is uncooperative, radiographs are essential.

There can be no hard and fast rules on the frequency of these tests. Radiographs are needed at specific intervals to determine pathological changes, such as resorption or periapical infections depending on the type of injuries sustained. As a general rule the following sequence of radiographs of injured teeth is a useful guide:

- *First visit.* Periapical, anterior occlusal, soft tissue views of lips (if needed), orthopantomogram (OPT) if indicated.
- *One month.* Further periapical or anterior occlusal views of damaged teeth. If root canal therapy (RCT) has been initiated, other working length views may be required.
- *Three months.* Further periapical views may be needed to check on periapical pathology or on the integrity of the root canal obturation.
- *Six months.* As for the three months assessment visit. Take periapical views. If several teeth are involved, an anterior occlusal film may be used.
- *Twelve months.* By this stage, in most cases, treatment of the trauma will either be entirely successful or it will not. Periapical radiographs will be indicated unless the case presents deteriorating periapical pathology or resorption. In these instances, periodic radiographs will still be required.
- *Subsequent years.* The frequency of further follow-up radiographs will be dependent on the type and extent of the trauma. In most cases this will be annually.

In some cases the trauma will be initially dealt with and there will be no further pathological changes evident. However, subsequently there can be breakdown of the surrounding tissues, the tooth may very slowly die and/or develop periapical infection; there may be further trauma which causes a new problem; there may be external or internal resorption starting. This last problem can occur years after the original injury.

When such changes occur, the frequency of taking radiographs reverts to the situation pertaining as for a new injury. In other words the problem is dealt with and then followed up at 3-, 6- and 12-month intervals or until the tooth or teeth concerned are stabilized and free of pathology.

The **radiographic views** to be taken in trauma cases will depend on the type of injury and the age and cooperation of the patient. The simplest classification for this is based on the dentitions: primary, mixed and permanent.

The **types of film** to be used will vary according to the view required. For small children, who have difficulty tolerating sharp film-holders in their mouths, the small size bitewing (size 0 periapical film) is very useful. It can be used instead of a standard periapical film.

The small bitewing can also be used to take an anterior occlusal view in a very small child.

A brief summary of the films and views to be taken is given below.

Primary teeth

- **Maxillary incisors**. Small periapical films (size 0), anterior occlusal views which can be taken with a standard film size or use a child-sized 0 film turned sideways.
- **Mandibular incisors**. These films not usually required, but a child-sized bitewing film may be used as a miniature anterior occlusal film.
- **Molars**. While it is very rare for primary molars to be traumatized, it does occur and periapical films are indicated or, in a child who has difficulty with intra-oral films, a bitewing.
- **Suspected facial fractures**. An OPT or other facial views, as are possible, bearing in mind the age of the child.

Mixed dentition

- **Maxillary incisors**. Individual periapical films, anterior occlusal views using a standard sized film or, if the child is small for their age, use a child-sized bitewing film turned sideways, as above.
- **Mandibular incisors**. Periapical films used as an anterior occlusal film.
- **Molars**. Injury to the primary molars may still occur, sometimes as a sports injury, for which periapical films are indicated or a bitewing.
- **Suspected facial fractures**. An OPT or other facial views as they are indicated.

Permanent teeth

- **Maxillary incisors**. Individual periapical films, anterior occlusal views using a standard-sized film if more than one incisor is involved.
- **Canines**. These are rarely injured, but if involved a separate periapical view is needed.
- **Premolars**. Again, rarely injured, but can be affected in some types of sports injury and periapical views are indicated.
- **Mandibular incisors**. Periapical films or an anterior occlusal film.
- **Molars**. Injury to the permanent molars may occur, sometimes as cuspal slicing injuries or cracked tooth as a sports injury, for which periapical films are indicated or a deep bitewing.

- **Suspected facial fractures**. An OPT or other facial views as they are indicated.

RADIOGRAPHIC TECHNIQUES

These techniques are for the most part standard procedures and the reader is referred to appropriate textbooks of dental radiology (Whaites, 1992). Alternatively, radiographic techniques suitable for children are described in several textbooks of paediatric dentistry (Bricker and Kasle, 1994; Curzon *et al.*, 1996). However, there are a number of variations of radiographic techniques, particularly for small children, which are useful for patients with traumatized teeth.

Small children

It is well known that infants often fall and damage their teeth during the period of toddling when they are learning to walk. These children present a problem to the dentist who needs to take a radiograph of the damaged tooth or teeth. The radiograph has, under most circumstances, to be taken (see Chapter 13), as it is necessary to determine root fractures, split teeth, alveolar fractures or suspected damage to the succedaneous teeth.

The technique is to use a small anterior occlusal view with the child being held on their mother's lap (Figure 2.1). The child is enclosed in the arms of their mother as shown. If the mother is pregnant, another adult – the dentist or dental nurse – could perfom this function. A small, child-sized, bitewing film is used (size 0), turned sideways, so as to function as an anterior occlusal film.

The parent should hold the child and the film. Both the child and parent face the same way, with the child's head being cradled against the parent's shoulder. The parent's left hand restrains the child's body and arms, while the right hand positions and holds the film. Alternatively, the parent's right hand stabilizes the head from the upward movement (to look at the X-ray machine head). The left hand then closes the lower jaw on the film (Figure 2.1b). The angulation of the X-ray cone to the film held in the child's mouth is shown in Figure 2.2.

The completed radiograph should show the crowns and roots of the primary incisors, as well as the developing crowns of the permanent incisors lying within the alveolar bone. A typical radiograph of a child's maxillary incisor teeth, showing a root fracture of tooth, is given in Figure 2.3.

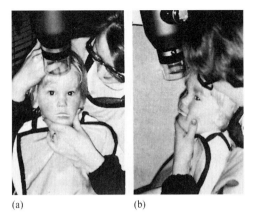

Figure 2.1 Parent and infant positioned for a maxillary anterior film using a size 0 bitewing: (a) anterior view; (b) lateral view

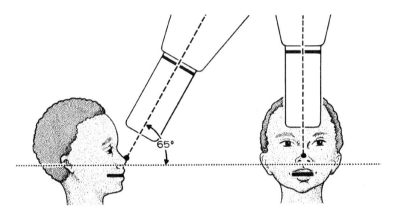

Figure 2.2 Anterior maxillary occlusal film using a small size 0 film. The cone is angled at +65 degrees and the central ray enters at the tip of the nose in the midline

If lower incisor teeth are involved, which is very rare in infants, a corresponding film in the lower arch is needed. The child's head is tilted upwards so that the occlusal plane is at 45 degrees to the horizontal. This correct head position is obtained by placing the X-ray cone at 25 degrees below the horizontal, the central ray being directed at the apices of the mandibular incisors. Completed radiographs should show the developing mandibular permanent incisors and the

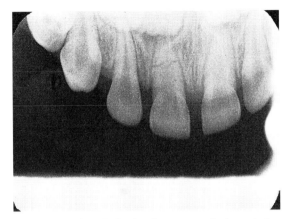

Figure 2.3 Radiograph showing the presence of primary incisor crowns and roots with developing crowns of permanent incisors. A fracture of tooth 51 is clearly seen

relationship of the primary incisor roots to these permanent crowns. Figure 2.4 shows a mandibular small size 0 film used as an anterior occlusal view in a small child.

Older children and adults

Older children, adolescents and young adults will not normally pose a problem for taking radiographs. In some cases, however, the shock of the trauma and the distress makes them unable to cooperate sufficiently for adequate radiographs to be taken. In these instances the dentist has to decide whether to force the issue and attempt a radiograph or to leave it until a later date when the patient may be

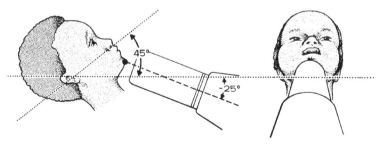

Figure 2.4 Mandibular anterior occlusal view using size 0 film to show primary incisors

more cooperative. The judgement to made here is to what degree the radiograph is essential.

The standard radiograph for the great majority of cases of dental trauma which involve maxillary incisors will be the periapical radiograph. A standard technique is described elsewhere (Whaites, 1992) and specifically for children by Curzon *et al.* (1996). If the lips are swollen or the teeth mobile, a gauze swab should be used to hold the film.

In most cases of trauma involving teeth, the lack of an immediate radiograph is not crucial. If there are doubts as to the presence of root fractures or luxations, the taking of a radiograph can be left to another appointment. Nevertheless radiographs *must* be taken in due course in order that all the necessary information for the proper long-term treatment of the patient is carried out. It is only in very rare cases that no radiographs are at all possible. In the latter instances adequate treatment planning cannot be carried out and it may also not be possible to provide even the most basic care without some form of sedation, relative analgesia or general anaesthetic. When this is the case, the general dental practitioner needs to refer the patient to a specialist unit.

SOFT TISSUE RADIOGRAPHS

During an accident involving damage to the teeth, fractures of the tooth substance often occur. In some cases the broken piece, or pieces, of tooth are lost or become imbedded in the soft tissues. Usually they are in the lips. As part of the initial diagnosis and treatment planning, questions need to be asked to determine the whereabouts of the missing piece(s) of tooth.

If it is not clear where the missing pieces of tooth are and there are cuts, lacerations or other damage to the lips, the dentist should be suspicious that they may be imbedded in the lips. To be absolutely sure, it is necessary to check by taking appropriate views of the lips. This is accomplished by having the patient hold an anterior occlusal film vertically alongside the face so that the radiographic beam passes through the lips to impinge on the film (Figure 2.5).

This view will also identify any other foreign bodies imbedded in the lips, such as soil or grit, as a result of the accident. These imbedded particles will show up on the radiograph as opaque materials (Figure 2.6). They will need to be removed by exploring the wound(s) after first providing local analgesia.

It is often a good idea to take further radiographs of this type after

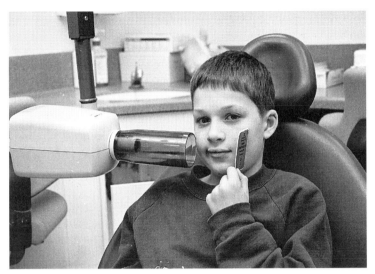

Figure 2.5 Photograph showing position of film to be used to take a radiograph of the lips to check for the presence of broken pieces of tooth

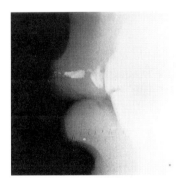

Figure 2.6 Radiograph of lips showing presence of pieces of a fractured tooth imbedded in the soft tissues

surgical intervention to make sure that all foreign particles have been removed.

STORING OF RADIOGRAPHS

An important consideration in the taking of radiographs for cases of dental trauma is the keeping of them. It is easy to just put the radiographs in the pocket of the standard dental record, but radiographs easily fall out and get lost. A better approach is to staple or stick them to a sheet of A4 size acetate. There are also commercially available mounting devices which may serve the purpose.

The aim of mounting all radiographs, and to do so chronologically, is first of all to make sure that they are not lost but secondly to enable them to be viewed simultaneously on an X-ray viewer. Changes over time can be much more readily seen by this approach.

SENSIBILITY TESTS

Sensibility tests, commonly referred to as 'vitality tests', are used to monitor the condition of the pulpal tissues of a traumatized tooth or teeth. They are essential to monitor the state of health of the pulpal nerve and blood vessels and to determine when a tooth is losing vitality. The tests use a number of approaches using either temperature, hot or cold, or electric pulp testing. It is advisable to use at least two methods and the usual sequence is a cold test with ethyl chloride followed by an electric test.

The techniques for sensibility testing are very straightforward and need little elaboration here. Cold testing with ethyl chloride is very simple. Electronic testing is more complicated and requires a full explanation to the patient before use. For younger children, the apparatus can be frightening.

The teeth to be tested should be cleaned gently, and dried. The reference electrode is placed on the patient's lip and a blob of contact gel is positioned on the centre of the facial surface of the tooth to be tested (Figure 2.7). The readings are taken sequentially and immediately recorded in Part IV of the trauma form (see Figure 1.2).

All test results need to be recorded on each visit (except the first) and this is often best accomplished using the trauma form. By making sure that all sensibility test results are recorded, any changes in vitality will become readily apparent as the recall visits progress.

First visit tests

Many experts feel that taking sensibility readings with tests on the visit of initial presentation are often not worth while. This is certainly so for complicated and complex traumas, such as severe luxations, etc. However, for uncomplicated injuries such as enamel or enamel–dentine chips it is important to record sensibility.

We cannot emphasize too strongly that the results of all sensibility tests should be carefully recorded on the trauma form. This means that there will always be an accurate record of the reactions of the

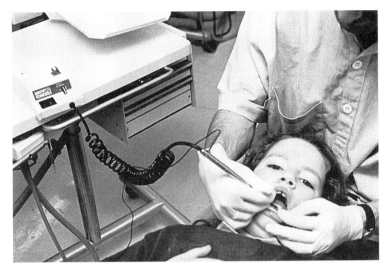

Figure 2.7 Photograph showing correct positioning of electrode for sensibility tests on mandibular teeth

pulps in affected teeth to tests. However, it also serves to record the continuing follow-up care that is being provided.

SUMMARY

Good-quality radiographs are absolutely essential to the management of dental trauma. The information given aids diagnosis and treatment planning for the care of traumatized teeth. Radiographs also serve to monitor changes in pulp and periapical conditions during the healing process. Similarly, after the first visit and initial shock to the teeth, sensibility tests need to be carried out routinely and the results meticulously recorded.

REFERENCES AND FURTHER READING

American Academy of Pediatric Dentistry (1993) *Guidelines for Prescribing Dental Radiographs.* American Academy of Pediatric Dentistry, Chicago
Bricker, S.L. and Kasle, M.J. (1994) Radiographic techniques. In *Dentistry for the Child and Adolescent,* 6th edn (edited by McDonald, R.E. and Avery, D.R.). Mosby, St Louis
Curzon, M.E.J., Roberts, J.F. and Kennedy, D.B. (1996) Radiographic techniques. In *Kennedy's Paediatric Operative Dentistry,* 4th edn. Butterworth-Heinemann, Oxford
Whaites, E. (1992) *Essentials of Dental Radiography and Radiology.* Churchill Livingstone, London

Chapter 3

Legal aspects: litigation and preparing legal reports

M.E.J. Curzon

Litigation is becoming more frequent as people are more inclined to seek redress for orofacial injuries. As mentioned in Chapter 1, this may occur some time after the injury and the dental practitioner will be required to provide a report for either plaintiff or defendant, or both, at some future date. This should be remembered when completing the dental records and emphasizes the use of the trauma form. Because there may be a long delay between treating a patient and preparing a report, the details written on the trauma form must always be legible. Dentists are encouraged to complete such a form slowly and with care, so that the notes can always be read. It is surprising how difficult it is, after a number of years, to read even one's own handwriting. Therefore, write clearly so that anybody will be able to read it at some time in the future. Any legal report that is required will be based on these dental notes.

PREPARATION OF LEGAL REPORTS

There is a way of preparing legal reports on dental trauma which has been developed over the years. Any dentist asked to prepare a report for the first time should take advice on the matter from someone with previous experience. Legal reports may appear to the novice in these matters a rather daunting task, but in fact are quite straightforward as long as the facts of the case are adhered to. What form should the report take? What should be included? Should it be entirely factual and when should the dentist make comments based on experience? Over the years there has grown up a depth of knowledge on style and presentation of legal reports which aids the dentist in knowing how to write them (Dental Protection, 1998).

Legal reports vary in type depending on the stage of the litigation and negotiations between the solicitors/lawyers of each party. Essentially reports are:

- **First report** – the initial statement describing the trauma and treatment to date.
- **Second report** – elaborating on the first report and giving an opinion as to extent of the injury, prognosis and possible outcome.
- **Quantum report** – assessing the financial costs of the trauma.
- **Liability and causation reports** – giving an opinion on these matters.
- **Final report** – which may be needed to cover any disputed aspects.

First report

The request for a legal report will come from a lawyer, usually a solicitor in the UK, saying that a case of trauma has resulted in there being a case whereby damages are being sought. The litigation concerning orofacial trauma will be brought on behalf of the traumatized patient, who is most often a minor and therefore on their behalf by a 'next friend', who is usually the parent or guardian.

Where the patient is older and of legal age, the case is brought by themselves. The dentist is identified in the solicitor's letter as the person who saw or treated the plaintiff and therefore a report on the injuries and subsequent treatment is needed.

Sometimes there is a request for a report on submitted documents where the defendant, that is the individual or agency being sued, is asking for information on a case in order to defend against the claim. The approach for the dentist who treated the patient suffering the trauma is, however, the same. A factual report on the diagnosis and treatment is required.

By following the formula described below, the preparation of the report becomes quite easy. This report is called the **first report** and is entirely factual. The first report should be written under the headings discussed below. The style should be simple, factual and not make unsupported statements. A dentist who receives a request for a report from a solicitor or lawyer should always ensure that there is a legal statement signed by the patient, or next best friend, authorizing the release of information from the patient's dental records.

1. *Credentials of the writer.* This simply states who the dentist is that is preparing the report, their status and qualifications.
2. *List of documents.* This is a list of the documents, if any, that the solicitor/lawyer has sent as part of the claim; it may also include the records of the dentist who treated the patient for the trauma. Their use is to assist in the compilation of the report. In some cases the dentist asked to write the report may not be the same one who treated the patient. The treating dentist's records should

indicate the dates, notes and treatments carried out. If the dentist providing treatment is asked to write the report, obviously it will be based only on that dentist's own records.

3. *History.* This records, in simple terms, what was the situation when the patient was first seen by the dentist, the diagnosis and treatment. Where there have been several visits these should be listed and commented on in chronological order. The wording should indicate what are the facts as recorded by the dentist based on the dental records (trauma form), photographs and radiographs. Where evidence is based upon the patient's, parent's or carer's, version of events (hearsay), this should be indicated by suitable wording such as '*the patient reported that the trauma was because they were hit in the mouth by a brick thrown by another child at school*'.

   As with any history, all background information pertinent to the case, such as medical and social history, should be recorded. Copies of these documents may be included with the report.

4. *Clinical examination and treatment.* Visits should be described in chronological order, detailing the clinical findings and treatment. All observations and comments should be objective. The report does not need to be excessively detailed but must record the salient facts.

5. *Radiographic report.* The report on the relevant radiographs should be entirely factual and not subjective. Thus, if there is evidence of internal or external resorption, the report should say where the resorption is and an approximation of its size. Comments that the resorption is increasing, or decreasing, are subjective and not warranted on the basis of one film. However, if there is a series of radiographs which do show a change, appropriate comments may be made.

6. *Photographs.* These days, with the wide availability of high-quality cameras, it is advantageous always to take photographs of orofacial trauma. If this is possible it is recommended that two pictures be taken of each view. At some time in the future it may be necessary to provide photographs for presentation in a court of law. In this case a reserve set of copies, for the dentist's own records, is essential. The report should note that photographs are available.

7. *Comments on documents.* Where documents, other than the dentist's own patient records, are included for the report, these need to be commented upon. Observations should, again, be entirely factual and objective. Comments can be made that there is missing information which, by the very nature of the trauma, should have been present. Similarly if normal clinical practice would have indicated that a radiograph(s) should have been taken and was/were not, then a comment to that effect is appropriate.

8. *Prognosis.* In many cases of orofacial trauma the dentist will be asked for an opinion on the prognosis for the damaged teeth. This may be asked for in a first report but is more often the subject of the second report. Where remedial treatment has been carried out, or is still under way, an indication of how successful this is likely to be should be given. Fortunately, after the extensive research studies of Andreassen and Andreassen (1994), the prognosis for many types of trauma to teeth and treatment outcomes under various circumstances can be given with some degree of reliability. Reference to this textbook and others, or published papers in the literature, can be used to support the dentist's assessment of likely prognosis. A dentist should be careful in making statements of prognosis and should ensure that, as far as possible, any prediction should be supported by scientific evidence based upon published research.

The completed first report is signed and dated. Obviously it is essential for a dentist to retain a copy of the report for future reference.

Further reports

A first report may be followed by a request for a **second report**, which may be subjective. In these instances the dentist is asked to express his or her interpretation of the clinical situation and/or records. In addition, the dentist may be asked to comment on the pain, suffering and discomfort that the patient has experienced. Sometimes, if treatment has been provided by another dentist, there may be a request to comment on whether the treatment was negligent or not. Such comments should only be based on the factual evidence and on the basis of standards of treatment that are usual and normal dental practice among general dental practitioners in the locality.

Quantum reports may be required subsequent to the first and second reports. Such a report requires the dentist to make an estimate as to the cost of treatment that will be needed for the foreseeable future. This can be quite difficult, as in many trauma cases the prognosis is uncertain and therefore there may be a number of treatment options that could occur.

For example, a child aged 8 years could have sustained a blow to a maxillary central incisor which involved a wide exposure of the pulp. Treatment was not provided until several hours after the damage occurred. The initial treatment was successful but, although over the next few months apex closure was attained, nevertheless lateral root resorption commenced. What is the prognosis and future treatment modalities for such a tooth? The resorption may stop and the tooth remain symptom free for many years, requiring only a permanent crown restoration. However, the resorption may also slowly progress and a root canal treatment may be required, eventually needing a post and crown. Perhaps the resorption may be unstoppable, so that ultimately the tooth could be lost. In that case will a partial upper denture be required (with replacements every so many years), or a bridge of some sort, or might there be the possibilities of an implant? All these options will have to be considered in a quantum report, with an appropriate realistic cost based on fees pertaining at the time of preparation of the report.

Liability and causation reports may be requested, dealing with the subjects indicated by their title. The writing of such reports should be approached with great caution, as a dentist is not usually in a position to comment on whether someone was liable for damages or whether they were responsible for the damage to the teeth.

This problem arises mostly where a third party might have been thought to be negligent, such as a local town council in not maintaining a footpath/pavement in good condition, so that a child trips over a stone, falls and breaks a tooth. In cases of assault it is also not usually within a dentist's responsibility. In the authors' experience, statements on liability should be avoided.

On the question of cause, a dentist should likewise be cautious. Any comments should be confined to statements of fact, for example that a tooth has been broken. The damage could have been by a blow and that the force to produce such an injury was likely to have been great. It is not in a dentist's area of expertise to speculate or comment on a likely cause.

Sometimes there be may be request for yet a further report (the **final report**) which will require comments on other documents being considered by the lawyers on both sides. In complex cases, all the documentation pertaining to a case may be submitted to a more senior lawyer with extensive experience in such cases for a learned opinion. In the UK, such senior lawyers are titled Queen's Counsellors (QC) and colloquially called 'silks'. Even in such an eventuality the dentist's role may not yet be over, as a request for a further report commenting on the silk's report may occur. As can be seen, the documentation in contested cases can become voluminous.

It is also clear that once litigation involving cases of orofacial trauma commences, the process may be long drawn out and take many years to resolve. In the authors' experience, such cases have taken four to five years before being settled or reaching a court of law for a judgement. In the latter case there will be a summons for the dentist who wrote the reports to appear in court as an expert witness.

It should be emphasized that an expert witness appears as a *counsel to the court* to help the court make a judgement on the merits of the case. They are rarely there to act on behalf of one side or the other. Should a dentist receive a summons to appear, they *must* attend. Not to do so is a contempt of court.

In the authors' experience, to actually have to appear in court is a very rare occurrence. It is not appropriate here to discuss appearing in court as, if it should occur, the expert witness will be counselled by the relevant lawyers as to how this is conducted. A reader of this book who is faced with such an eventuality is strongly encouraged to read an excellent book on this particular aspect of being an expert witness (Medical Protection Society, 1995). In addition, expert advice can be obtained from the dentist's own protection society.

A word of caution

It must be emphasized that on occasion an expert witness may be asked to alter a report, and it is important that a dentist does not make changes to the point where it would affect their own credibility. This is particularly important in assault cases, as noted above, where the expert might be led to go beyond his or her remit by commenting on likely causation. In these circumstances it becomes very easy for a barrister/lawyer on the opposite side (usually the defence) to destroy the credibility of the expert witness (the dentist).

SUMMARY

Dentists will increasingly be required to provide legal reports concerning dental trauma. Good documentation of each and every patient treated for trauma will ensure that when a request for a legal report arrives the necessary detailed information is at hand. The preparation of legal reports is straightforward so long as the formal processes, outlined here, are followed.

REFERENCES AND FURTHER READING

Andreasen, J.O. and Andreasen, F.M. (1994) *Textbook and Colour Atlas of Traumatic Injuries to the Teeth*. Munksgaard, Copenhagen

Dental Protection (1998) *Second Opinions, Reports and Expert Evidence*. Dental Protection, London

Medical Protection Society (1995) *Medico-legal Reports and Appearing in Court*. The Medical Protection Society, London

Smith, B.G.N. (1997) *Writing Expert Reports*, Information Spotlight. Dental Protection, London

Smith, B.G.N. (1997) *Writing Dento-legal Reports as 'Expert'*, Information Spotlight. Dental Protection, London

Chapter 4

Uncomplicated crown fractures: infractions, enamel fractures and enamel–dentine fractures

K.J. Toumba

Crown fractures of permanent teeth occur in about 75% of all tooth fractures (Andreasen and Andreasen, 1994). Recent research has shown that when treatment is delayed, even for only a few hours or days, the prognosis is poor (Hamilton *et al.*, 1997). The prognosis is good when these cases are treated as emergencies and restorations placed immediately. This chapter will therefore cover the definition, aetiology, diagnosis, clinical recognition, treatment, review and prognosis for teeth that have sustained either an infraction, enamel fracture or uncomplicated enamel–dentine fracture following dental trauma.

Definitions

- **Infractions**. Minor and incomplete fractures (crazes or cracks) of the enamel with or without loss of tooth substance.
- **Enamel fractures**. Fractures with loss of tooth substance confined to the enamel (uncomplicated crown fracture).
- **Enamel–dentine fractures**. Fractures with loss of tooth substance confined to enamel and dentine but not involving the pulp (uncomplicated crown fracture).

INFRACTIONS

Aetiology

Enamel infractions are very common and account for 10.5–12.5% of acutely traumatized incisors (Ravn, 1981a), but are frequently overlooked. Infractions are commonly caused by traumatic injuries to the permanent dentition and seem to be rare or unknown in the primary dentition. They usually occur following the direct impact of a force to the teeth, and may appear with or without loss of tooth structure (although infractions most frequently occur without loss of tooth substance). Infraction lines presenting on posterior teeth are usually implicated in the 'cracked tooth syndrome' and not associated with dental trauma.

Pathology

Enamel infractions appear as dark lines running parallel to the enamel rods and terminate at the dentino-enamel junction when ground sections of enamel are examined under the microscope.

Diagnosis and clinical recognition

Infraction lines appear as crazing or cracking within the enamel which do not cross the dentino-enamel junction and are best seen when the tooth is transilluminated. This can easily be achieved by the use of a curing light. Typically, infraction lines are described as horizontal, vertical or diagonal. It is very easy to overlook infractions using direct illumination, but they are easily visualized with transillumination using a fibreoptic light beam directed to shine through the tooth.

The tip of the light is placed lingually behind the tooth so that the light shines through the crown of the tooth (Figure 4.1).

Various pattern types of infraction lines can often be seen, depending on the direction of the impacting force and the location site on the tooth surface where the impact was made. Infraction lines may be the only evidence of trauma, and their presence should alert the clinician to the possible damage of the pulp and supporting dental structures, which should be evaluated carefully.

Treatment

Usually infractions do not require any definitive treatment. Sometimes, if there are sensitivity problems because of fluids leaking down the crack to the dentine, it is necessary to coat the crown with clear sealant or bonding agent, described below.

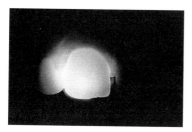

Figure 4.1 Photograph of a maxillary incisor transilluminated to show an infraction

Radiographs – two periapical radiographs at differing angulations (15 degrees)

These radiographs should be taken to determine the extent of any associated injury to the supporting dental structures (e.g. to eliminate the possibility of root fracture) and to serve as a baseline record for future follow-up.

Sensibility tests – assessment of tooth vitality as a baseline reading

Because it is uncertain whether the infraction line will stop short of the dentine or pulp, sensibility testing should be carried out to assess pulp vitality on presentation and to give baseline data for future follow-up. This should be performed by comparison with adjacent or contralateral teeth. Teeth with infractions limited to enamel will respond positively at the time of injury and remain positive to future testing. If the response is negative at the time of injury, endodontic therapy is not indicated immediately, but should be delayed until the patient develops symptoms associated with a necrotic pulp or there is radiographic evidence of periapical pathology.

Use of sealants – seal infraction lines with unfilled resin

Sealing of infraction lines with unfilled resins using an acid etch technique may be indicated. This will prevent the uptake of stains from foods, drinks and tobacco smoking (e.g. tea, coffee, cola, red wine, chlorhexidine mouthwashes, and tobacco products).

Warning

If the infraction line is deep and runs through to the dentine in an immature tooth, there may be pain on etching of the tooth. The acid will easily penetrate to the dento-enamel junction, causing a pulpal response. Care should be taken here and it is recommended that an acid gel be used, but only for a brief period of time, about 15 seconds, sufficient to allow the enamel to be etched to enable the fissure sealant material to adhere to the enamel.

Review appointments

Patients should be reviewed to follow up the affected teeth at the following times:

- 6–8 weeks;
- 3 months;
- 6 months;
- yearly for 3 years.

At these times, sensibility testing should be performed and radiographs taken. The latter should be at the 3-month and yearly follow-up appointments.

Prognosis

The prognosis of enamel infractions, if treated promptly, is excellent. The risk of pulp necrosis is extremely small. Ravn (1981a) reported that 3.5% of 1337 incisors suffering from enamel infractions and followed up for at least two years, resulted in pulp death. The small group of teeth that became necrotic were possibly due to overlooked concussion or luxation injuries that occurred at the same time as the infraction injury.

Infractions – summary of treatment approach

- Take full trauma **history** using trauma form.
- Take periapical **radiographs**.
- Record **sensibility** tests and results.
- Place fissure **sealant(s)** to protect tooth/teeth.
- Routine **follow-up** at 6 weeks, 3, 6 and 12 months, then yearly.

ENAMEL FRACTURES

Aetiology

Crown fractures in the permanent dentition account for 26–76% of dental injuries and 4–38% in the primary dentition (Andreasen and Ravn, 1972). Crown fractures of primary teeth are rare, owing to the soft, resilient nature of the supporting structures.

A portion of the tooth enamel is lost following an injury when the impact force is directed either perpendicular or obliquely to the incisal edge of the tooth. The most common aetiological factors for injuries to the permanent dentition are falls (usually involving bicycles, skate boards or during icy conditions), contact sports (especially rugby, hockey, judo and karate), road traffic accidents, foreign bodies (such as missiles, cricket bats or balls, bottles, stones, etc.) or due to altercations (especially fighting in boys). Injuries of this nature predominantly occur in boys rather than girls. However, injuries sustained from horse-riding or swimming accidents seem to occur more frequently with girls.

Clinical recognition

Crown fractures without pulpal involvement occur more frequently than complicated crown fractures (Andreasen and Ravn, 1972). They are usually confined to a single tooth (invariably the maxillary central incisors) and the fracture usually involves the mesial or distal corners of the incisors.

However, there are many ways in which crown fractures may present. Isolated enamel fractures do not usually compromise pulp health, but are generally irritating to the soft tissues (especially the tongue and lips) and pose an aesthetic concern to the patient.

Diagnosis

The diagnosis of the various forms of non-complicated crown fracture is straightforward. As with all aspects of trauma the first step, even for very minor crown fractures, is the completion of a trauma form, as described in Chapter 1. Once this is completed, the patient should then have the appropriate radiographs taken. This is necessary because, while a crown fracture may appear to be non-complicated, there is always the risk that there may have been associated root fractures as well. Similarly, sensibility tests are also required.

There is not a great urgency to start intervention and restorative care for these cases and therefore the diagnostic tests can be interspersed between the care of other patients. Thus once the trauma form has been initially completed, the patient with this type of trauma may be left for a time. The radiographs can be taken and another patient attended to while they are being developed. Again, the sensibility tests can be carried out in between seeing other patients.

The diagnosis of non-complicated injuries must preclude the presence of other complicating injuries. Then the treatment of the injury can proceed.

Treatment

Fractures limited to the enamel are treated by either recontouring the traumatized tooth or by restoring the missing portion of tooth enamel with a dental composite material.

Radiographs – two periapical radiographs at differing angulations (15 degrees)

These should be taken to determine the extent of any associated injury to the supporting dental structures (e.g. to eliminate the possibility of root fracture) and to serve as a baseline record for future follow-up. The size of the pulp and the stage of root development can also be assessed.

Sensibility tests – sensibility testing should be carried out to assess pulp vitality

In the case of simple enamel fractures, sensibility tests are needed on presentation and to provide baseline data for future follow-up. This should be performed by comparison with adjacent or contralateral teeth.

If the response is negative at the time of injury, endodontic therapy is not indicated immediately, but should be delayed until the patient develops symptoms associated with a necrotic pulp or there is radiographic evidence of periapical pathology.

Recontouring – injured tooth/teeth should be recontoured

If the enamel fracture is very small ($<$ 2 mm), the crown can be recontoured using either sandpaper discs in a slow-speed handpiece or with fine diamond burs in a high-speed air turbine handpiece. Occasionally it may also be necessary to recontour adjacent teeth. Where dentine has been exposed, no matter how small, this approach should not be used.

An enamel fracture involving the distal incisal corner may be recontoured to accentuate the rounded edge, but a similarly involved mesial corner fracture will require restoration rather than recontouring in order to maintain the aesthetic appearance. In a young patient, where the permanent incisors have only recently erupted, it may be necessary to recontour an incisor to reproduce the mamelons.

Composite and adhesive resin restorations – replace missing tooth structure

Missing tooth structure should be replaced with composite resin using an acid etch composite technique (Figure 4.2). The tooth is cleaned and air dried and an acid etchant (37% phosphoric acid) applied to the affected portion to produce microporosities in the enamel surface. Unfilled resin is applied as a bonding agent and cured (usually light

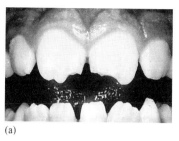 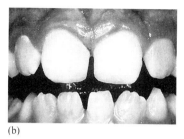

(a)   (b)

Figure 4.2 Photograph of a maxillary incisor (11) with an enamel fracture restored with composite resin: (a) fractured 11 and 21; (b) restored incisors (11 enamel fracture, 21 enamel–dentine fracture)

cured) to create interlocking tags and a suitable shade of composite resin material is applied and cured. As enamel fractures are usually small, the composite material may be applied 'freehand' and contoured after curing.

Review appointments

Patients should be reviewed to follow up the affected teeth at the following times:

- 6–8 weeks;
- 3 months;
- 6 months;
- yearly for 3 years.

At these times, sensibility testing should be performed and periapical radiographs taken. This is important because teeth with minor fractures may suffer concussion and their pulp tissues slowly die over many months.

Prognosis

The prognosis of enamel fractures is good. Ravn (1981b) reported that 1.7% of 2891 permanent incisors, suffering from enamel fractures as the only damage, resulted in pulpal necrosis. The risk of pulp canal obliteration has been reported to be 0.5% and for root resorption to be 0.2%. Irrespective of which treatment option is selected to treat enamel fractures, the procedure must be performed immediately to prevent any potential drifting, tilting or over-eruption of adjacent and opposing teeth.

ENAMEL–DENTINE FRACTURES

Aetiology

The aetiological factors for enamel–dentine fracture are identical to those for enamel fractures described earlier. It is *important to treat and restore these fractures immediately*. They should not be left with unprotected dentine to a later appointment. Contamination of the dentine will occur and pulp death may well ensue.

Diagnosis and clinical recognition

Uncomplicated crown fracture involving enamel and dentine occurs more frequently than any other type of crown injury in the permanent dentition. They need to be treated quickly and effectively and not left. This is because there is usually a wide exposure of the dentine which is easily contaminated by dirt, oral fluids, food and bacteria.

The clinical examination of fractured teeth should include the following:

- Thorough **cleansing** of the injured teeth with a water spray.
- **Assessment** of the extent of exposed dentine.
- Evaluation of **thermal and masticatory sensitivity**.
- Check whether the **dental pulp** is visible under a thin layer of dentine.
- **Sensibility testing** (as described earlier).
- **Radiographic examination** (as described earlier).

Treatment

Treatment should be carried out considering:

- the immediate needs of the patient (emergency versus definitive care);
- the pulpal response to the injury;
- the effect of the restorative materials on the pulp;
- the definitive restorative treatment option.

The missing tooth structure should be replaced immediately to prevent the possible unwanted sequelae of:

- labial protrusion;
- drifting or tilting of adjacent teeth;
- over-eruption of opposing teeth;
- bacterial contamination of dentine and pulp.

The treatment options for restoration of enamel–dentine fractures are:

- composite adhesive resin restoration;
- reattachment of the original tooth fragment;
- laminate veneers;
- porcelain fused to metal crowns;
- full-coverage porcelain jacket crowns.

Liners

There is some controversy as to whether liners should or should not be used for acid-etched resin restorations. In summary, the points of controversy are:

- There is evidence that calcium hydroxide cements disintegrate both during the acid etching procedure and beneath restorations with time.
- Bacteria have been found within calcium hydroxide used as liners (Cox *et al.*, 1985), thus rendering the restoration susceptible to microleakage.
- Calcium hydroxide liners have been demonstrated to have the same softening effect on composite resins as zinc oxide–eugenol liners (Reinhardt and Chalkey, 1983).
- Hydrophilic liners are superior to hydrophobic liners in sealing the dentinal tubules.
- Sealing of the dentinal tubules and thus protection from bacterial and restorative irritants appears to be a critical factor in pulp healing.
- Adequately sealed exposed dentine will form reparative dentine even without calcium hydroxide (Andreasen and Andreasen, 1994).
- Glass ionomer cements (e.g. Vitrebond[R]) are preferable to calcium hydroxide as liners to seal the dentinal tubules.
- For exposed dentine within 2 mm of the pulp, a thin layer of calcium hydroxide is still recommended, followed by coverage with a glass ionomer cement (e.g. Vitrebond[R]).

Composite and adhesive resin restorations

The majority of teeth with enamel–dentine fractures are restored using composite resin materials. This can be performed:

- 'freehand';
- using a cellulose acetate crown former;
- by taking an alginate impression and obtaining a laboratory-made

crown former (this is particularly useful for restoring multiple crown fractures).

Many clinicians do not perform any enamel preparation, in order to minimize removal of sound tooth structure. However, despite the improvement in bond strengths of modern resin-bonded materials, loss of the restoration can occur (see Chapter 12). This is more likely to occur with smaller fractures, as the strength of the enamel–resin bond is weaker.

Hence, enamel preparation may be indicated in certain situations. This can be achieved by creating a 'chamfer-shoulder' preparation that has a length of 2 mm and a depth of one-half the thickness of enamel. Alternatively, the finish line can be a bevel preparation along the length of the fracture. The advantage of definite finishing lines is that a better aesthetic result is achieved by elimination of the demarcation between the composite resin and the tooth.

Technique

The technique is straightforward and is described below and also in Chapter 12:

- **Clinical assessment** and diagnosis.
- Administer **local analgesia** if required.
- **Clean** fractured tooth by gentle water spray irrigation.
- Select **shade** of composite material.
- **Rubber dam** isolation.
- Apply a **liner** (glass ionomer is preferable to calcium hydroxide) to exposed dentine.
- **Enamel preparation** ('bevel' or 'chamfer-shoulder' preparations if indicated).
- **Etch** enamel for 30 seconds using 37% phosphoric acid.
- **Wash** with water.
- Thoroughly **air dry**.
- Apply dentine **bonding agent** and restore tooth to original contour with selected composite material.
- **Cure** composite resin thoroughly.
- **Contour** and finish margins with sandpaper discs and/or diamond/carbide finishing burs.
- **Polish** restoration.
- **Check occlusion**.

Successful restorations of enamel–dentine fractures using composite resin can last for many years (see Figure 12.1). The key to success is not to rush the restoration but to carry it out with meticulous attention to maintaining a dry field, proper tooth cleaning, complete etching, thorough washing and drying and the necessary curing time. In a very busy schedule it is in the patient's best interest that temporary coverage of the exposed dentine is performed, perhaps with a bonding agent such as Vitrebond^R, and then for the patient to be booked in for a separate visit at which a definitive restoration can be placed.

Reattachment of crown fragment

It is quite possible to reattach the broken crown of a tooth (Figure 4.3). This approach is successful in the short term but may require restorative procedures on subsequent occasions. In the authors' experience it is not very easy to do, but if successful gives a very good result. The problems with the technique are moisture and crevicular fluid control. In attempting to bond the tooth crown back into place it has to be accurately located to its original position, at the same time ensuring that there is no contamination of the broken tooth surfaces. Any moisture at the wrong time means that the bonding agents do not work and inadequate adhesion ensues.

This approach requires isolation of the affected tooth or teeth using a rubber dam. The broken piece of crown is then trial fitted to ensure that it will still go back into place. The greatest difficulty is maintaining the exposed enamel and dentine surfaces completely dry, because of gingival fluid oozing around the neck of the tooth. Sometimes there has been soft tissue damage, and bleeding causes contamination of the enamel and/or dentine. This approach is always worth a try, but in the authors' experience it is more economic in time to proceed directly to a composite resin restoration.

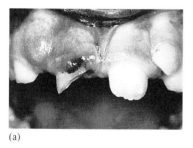
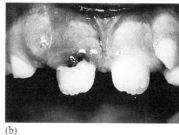

(a)   (b)

Figure 4.3 Photograph of fractured incisor restored with crown fragment bonded back into place: (a) fractured tooth 11; (b) fragment reattached

Technique

- Clinical **assessment** and diagnosis.
- Check the **fit of the fragment**.
- **Clean** fragment and tooth with a pumice-water slurry.
- **Select shade** of composite material.
- **Rubber dam** isolation.
- **Attach fragment** to a piece of gutta-percha or sticky wax to facilitate handling.
- **Etch** enamel for 30 seconds on both fracture surfaces using 37% phosphoric acid.
- **Wash** with water and air dry.
- Apply **dentine bonding** agent to both surfaces and cure.
- Place **composite resin** over both surfaces and position fragment, remove excess.
- **Cure** both labially and palatally for 60 seconds.
- **Remove** a 1 mm **gutter of enamel** on each side of the entire fracture line to a depth of 0.5 mm using a small round diamond bur.
- **Etch** the newly prepared enamel, wash, dry, apply composite, and cure (this will reinforce the strength of the fragment).
- **Contour** and finish margins with sandpaper discs and/or diamond/carbide finishing burs.
- **Polish** restoration.
- **Check occlusion**.

Other restorative options

- Laminate veneers.
- Porcelain fused to metal crowns.
- Full-coverage porcelain jacket crowns.

The majority of crown fractures are restored using composite resin materials. Therefore, these alternative restorative techniques should usually only be considered (if indicated) when the patient has attained full maturity and development of the dental arches. This occurs at about 16 years of age. The reasoning behind this is that there is continued eruption of the teeth until after puberty has passed. This continued eruption means that if a laminate veneer or crown is placed on a young tooth then, within a few months, the continued eruption of the tooth, usually a maxillary incisor, exposes the neck of the tooth. This shows as a dark line at the gingival margin and is aesthetically unacceptable. As these advanced restorations are expensive their use should be delayed until all growth and eruption of the teeth has ceased.

Review appointments

As discussed before, patients should be reviewed to follow up the affected teeth at the following times:

- 6–8 weeks;
- 3 months;
- 6 months;
- yearly for 3 years.

At these times, sensibility testing should be performed and radiographs taken.

Prognosis

Ravn (1981c) reported that 3.2% of 3144 permanent incisors suffering from enamel–dentine fractures, as the only damage, resulted in pulpal necrosis. Ravn's study also showed that factors such as associated luxation injuries, the stage of root development, the type of treatment received and the extent of the dentine exposed, exerted significant influence upon the risk of pulp necrosis. His study also showed that, for deep fractures, pulp necrosis occurred in 54% of untreated teeth and in only 8% of treated teeth. This emphasizes the importance of performing immediate restoration of crown-fractured teeth and the need to treat these traumatized teeth as emergencies.

SUMMARY

Uncomplicated dental trauma occurring as infractions, enamel chips and enamel–dentine fractures are very straightforward to deal with. They should never be left untreated and coverage of any exposed dentine is immediately needed. The follow-up of these cases with radiographic and sensibility tests is essential as these teeth can still become non-vital even though the trauma seems to be minor.

REFERENCES AND FURTHER READING

Andreasen, J.O. and Andreasen, F.M. (1994) *Textbook and Colour Atlas of Traumatic Injuries to the Teeth*, 3rd edn. Munksgaard, Copenhagen

Andreasen, J.O. and Ravn, J.J. (1972) Epidemiology of traumatic dental injuries to primary and permanent teeth in a Danish population sample. *International Journal of Oral Surgery*, **1**, 235–239

Cox, C.F., Bergenholtz, G., Heys, D.R., Syed, S.A., Fitzgerald, M. and Heys, R.J. (1985) Pulp capping of dental pulp mechanically exposed to oral microflora: a 1–2 year observation of wound healing in the monkey. *Journal of Oral Pathology*, **14**, 156–168

Hamilton, F.A., Hill, F.J. and Holloway, P.J. (1997) An investigation of dento-alveolar trauma and its treatment in an adolescent population. Part 1 and 2. *British Dental Journal*, **182**, 91–95, 129–133

Ravn, J.J. (1981a) Follow-up study of permanent incisors with enamel cracks as a result of an acute trauma. *Scandinavian Journal of Dental Research*, **89**, 117–123

Ravn, J.J. (1981b) Follow-up study of permanent incisors with enamel fractures as a result of an acute trauma. *Scandinavian Journal of Dental Research*, **89**, 213–217

Ravn, J.J. (1981c) Follow-up study of permanent incisors with enamel–dentin fractures as a result of an acute trauma. *Scandinavian Journal of Dental Research*, **89**, 355–365

Reinhardt, J.W. and Chalkey, Y. (1983) Softening effects of bases on composite resins. *Clinical Preventive Dentistry*, **5**, 9–12

Roberts, G.F. and Longhurst, P. (1996) *Oral and Dental Trauma in Children and Adolescents*. University Press, Oxford

Chapter 5

Complicated crown fractures: fractures of the crown involving the pulp

M.S. Duggal

When the trauma results in the fracture of a crown, exposing the pulp (Figure 5.1), bacterial contamination of the pulp tissue will occur at the exposure site. Therefore, the time interval between injury and treatment is the key to successful management. The treatment provided should either seal off the pulp from further contamination or effectively eradicate the contaminated tissue as soon as possible, in order to allow the rest of the pulp to heal.

RATIONALE OF TREATMENT

In teeth with incomplete root development and/or open apices, it is most important to maintain pulp vitality so that the root development can continue. If the tooth were to become non-vital, the root development would cease immediately with serious consequences for endodontic management (Figure 5.2). For teeth with open apices, therefore, treatment efforts should be directed to maintaining the vitality of the pulp in order to allow the normal processes of root-end closure (apexogenesis) to continue.

In teeth where the root development is complete, the important consideration is to maintain the tooth in an infection-free state. If severe contamination has occurred and the pulp has to be extirpated, a good root filling can easily be carried out to achieve this aim.

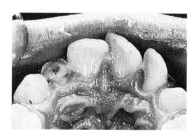

Figure 5.1 Fracture of a right maxillary lateral incisor showing exposure of pulp tissue

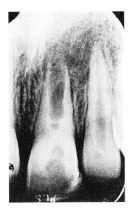

Figure 5.2 Radiograph showing arrested development of the root of tooth 21 due to trauma

DIAGNOSIS AND CONSIDERATIONS FOR TREATMENT PLANNING

When a patient presents with a fracture of the crown that has exposed the pulp, the following factors should be considered before the choice of treatment is made.

Clinical

- Size of exposure.
- Degree of contamination.
- Time elapsed since exposure.

These factors are important because of the greater risk of bacterial contamination of larger exposures once exposed to the salivary micro-organisms for prolonged periods. The prognosis for pulp healing for a small pulp exposure in a patient who has sought treatment soon after the injury is excellent. In such a case, because of minimal contamination, a conservative procedure such as a direct pulp capping would be adequate, as opposed to a more radical treatment modality such as a pulpotomy. The latter would be required where there are larger pulp exposures which have been contaminated for some time.

Radiographic

The radiograph(s) are used to assess the stage of root development. As discussed before, the stage of the root development is one of the most critical factors that will determine the final treatment plan in younger children. A good periapical radiograph is therefore required before any treatment is planned.

THERAPEUTIC METHODS FOR TREATMENT OF TRAUMATICALLY EXPOSED PULPS

Three techniques are available for treating exposed pulps:

1. **Direct pulp capping**.
2. **Pulpotomy**:
   - Partial pulpotomy (Cvek's technique)
   - Full coronal pulpotomy.
3. **Pulpectomy**:
   - Immediate obturation with gutta-percha
   - Apexification followed by obturation.

The methods to be used are:

Direct pulp capping

Indicated for pulp exposures that are:

- very small (pinpoint) (Figure 5.3);
- recent;
- not grossly contaminated.

Clinical technique

- **Cover the exposed pulp** with hard setting calcium hydroxide (Dycal^R) (Figure 5.4).
- Apply a further layer of glass ionomer based material over the calcium hydroxide to provide a **leak-proof seal**.
- **Build the tooth** up using one of the methods described in Chapter 12.

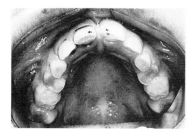

Figure 5.3 Fracture of maxillary left central incisor with a pinpoint (<2 mm) exposure suitable for pulp capping as long as the exposure time has been less than one hour

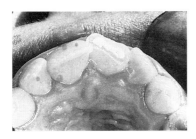

Figure 5.4 Photograph of exposed pulp in a fractured incisor after pulp capping with Dycal[R]

Whenever possible, a full-coverage restoration of the crown with composite resin should be carried out, as this ensures that no further contamination of the pulp can occur. It is tempting in a busy dental practice to place an intermediate dressing such as a glass ionomer cement and to recall the patient for a final restoration. It is the authors' experience that many such dressings are not secure and will come off, allowing pulp contamination to occur, compromising the pulp prognosis.

The success rate of direct pulp capping for small traumatic exposure, where there is no concomitant luxation, is excellent if carried out promptly and as described above.

Pulpotomy

Depending on the size of the pulp exposure and the degree of contamination, amputation of the pulp can be carried out at different levels. Two techniques are usually described – partial and coronal.

Partial pulpotomy

This procedure was first described by Cvek (1978) and is also referred to as *Cvek's technique.*

Rationale

The spread of inflammation through the dental pulp due to the invading micro-organisms is slow, as the pulp has well-developed defence mechanisms. Therefore, for contaminated exposures, exposed for some time (several days old), where a direct pulp capping would not be appropriate, the removal of 2–4 mm of pulp tissue from around the exposure site would remove most of the infected pulp, leaving behind healthy tissue. The aim is to remove all possibly infected tissue and replace it with calcium hydroxide which then stimulates repair of the pulp with a secondary dentine bridge.

Indications

- Larger than a pinpoint exposure (Figure 5.5).
- Up to 4 days old.
- Teeth with complete or incomplete root development.

Clinical technique

- Use **local analgesia** and apply a rubber dam.
- **Enlarge** the exposure with a high-speed handpiece and a diamond bur so that the cavity is about 2–4 mm wide (Figure 5.6a).
- Using small sharp excavators **remove pulp tissue** only from the area that has been accessed with the bur (2–4 mm around exposure).
- Dip a small **cotton pledget in saline** and place over the amputation site. Leave for 4–5 minutes until the bleeding stops.
- Place non-hard setting **calcium hydroxide** (Hypocal^R) over the pulp once the bleeding has stopped.
- Place a further layer of **glass ionomer** cement (Vitrebond^R) over the calcium hydroxide, providing a leak-proof lining and preventing further contamination.
- **Restore** the crown with composite resin (Figure 5.6b).

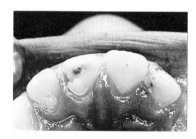

Figure 5.5 Larger exposure of the pulp of a fractured maxillary right central incisor where a partial pulpotomy is indicated

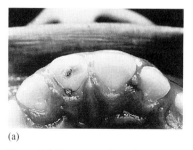

(a)

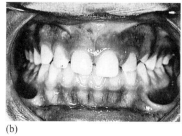

(b)

Figure 5.6 Treatment of a pulp exposure by the Cvek technique: (a) enlarge the exposure with a high-speed handpiece and a diamond bur so that the cavity is about 2–4 mm wide; (b) the tooth restored with composite resin

Follow-up

Both clinical and radiographic follow-up is required every 3 months for the first year and 6-monthly in the second year. Once pulp amputation, however minimal, has been carried out, pulp sensibility tests should not be relied upon as sole indicators of continued pulp vitality.

The following are the indicators of success:

Clinical

- Absence of any pain or discomfort from the tooth.
- Normal colour of the crown.
- No evidence of an abscess, e.g. sinus.

Radiographic

- No evidence of any periapical pathology on periapical radiographs.
- Evidence of continued root development, in cases where the root development was incomplete (Figure 5.7).

The partial pulpotomy technique is extremely useful and should be in the repertoire of all dentists who are called upon to treat complicated crown fractures in young children. The technique is usually described for the teeth where the root development is not yet complete and the continued vitality of the pulp tissue is critical. There is no reason, however, for it not to be used in the management of

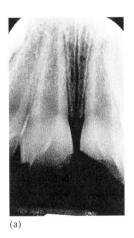

(a)

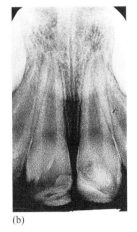

(b)

Figure 5.7 Radiographs showing continued root development after a Cvek procedure: (a) preoperative radiograph; (b) postoperative radiograph taken 8 months later showing continued root development of teeth 11 and 21

small, uncontaminated exposures in adolescents and adults as the least radical option. Success rates in excess of 95% have been reported for this technique (Fuks *et al.*, 1987), irrespective of the stage of root development.

Coronal pulpotomy

Coronal pulpotomy is indicated in large and contaminated exposures, but only in those cases where the root development is incomplete or the apex is wide open. With this technique the whole of the coronal pulp tissue is amputated, preserving non-inflamed vital pulp in the root canal, thus allowing continued root development.

Indications

- Teeth with incomplete root development only.
- Larger than a pinpoint exposure.
- Contaminated exposure site or more than 4 days old.

Clinical technique

- Use **local analgesia** and apply a rubber dam.
- **Enlarge the exposure** with a high-speed handpiece and a diamond bur so that access can be gained to the entire pulp chamber (Figure 5.8).
- With small sharp excavators **remove pulp tissue** from the entire coronal pulp chamber up to the cervical constriction, taking care to remove tissue from the pulp horns.
- Failure to remove pulp remnants from the pulp horns might lead to eventual discoloration of the crown with consequences for aesthetics.

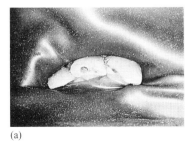 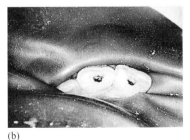

(a)   (b)

Figure 5.8 Photograph showing enlargement of an exposure with bur: (a) large exposure; (b) enlargement of exposure

- Dip a small **cotton pledget in saline** and place over the amputation site, and leave for 4–5 minutes until the bleeding stops.
- Place non-hard setting **calcium hydroxide** (Hypocal[R]) over the pulp once the bleeding has stopped (Figure 5.9); if the bleeding is not easily arrested, the root canal tissue is likely to be irreversibly inflamed and would require complete extirpation.
- Place a further layer of **glass ionomer** cement (Vitrebond[R]) over the calcium hydroxide to provide a leak-proof lining preventing further contamination.
- **Restore** the crown with composite resin (Figure 5.10).

Follow-up

Both clinical and radiographic follow-up, as described for the partial pulpotomy technique, should be carried out. In cases where coronal pulpotomy has been successfully carried out, a hard tissue layer just apical to the amputation site and continued root development can usually be demonstrated on the follow-up periapical radiographs (Figure 5.11).

Prognosis

The success rate for teeth treated with a coronal pulpotomy is modest (no more than 75%), compared with those treated with the partial pulpotomy technique. There is also an increased incidence of pulp canal obliteration in teeth that have been treated with a radical

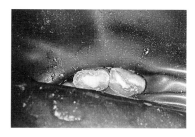

Figure 5.9 Non-hard setting calcium hydroxide placed over pulp exposure

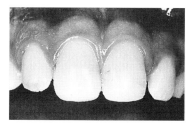

Figure 5.10 Restoration of maxillary incisor after a pulpotomy technique with composite resin

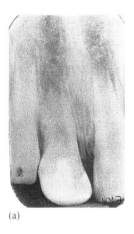

(a)

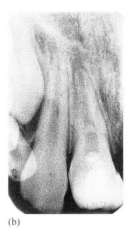

(b)

Figure 5.11 Periapical follow-up radiograph of maxillary incisor treated with a calcium hydroxide pulpotomy technique: (a) immediate postoperative radiograph showing incomplete root development; (b) continued root development after 12 months

pulpotomy (Figure 5.12). There is debate in the literature whether to regard the coronal pulpotomy technique as a definitive procedure or only a means to achieve root development. It has been suggested that due to the lower success rate with this technique, and also an increased risk of pulp canal obliteration, once the root development has been achieved, the root canal should be re-accessed, the remaining pulp extirpated and obturation done with gutta-percha. In the authors' opinion, pulp canal obliteration is not an indication for root canal treatment. It has been shown convincingly in the literature that fewer than 10% of those teeth that have undergone such a change are at risk

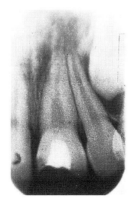

Figure 5.12 Radiograph showing obliteration of root canal previously treated with a radical pulpotomy

of becoming non-vital. Such teeth can be treated with a surgical approach, with retrograde filling.

Coronal pulpotomy should be regarded as a definitive procedure and no further treatment should be required unless, of course, any complications develop.

Pulpectomy

This technique is for cases where there is gross contamination of pulp or where the time lapse between the injury and a patient seeking treatment renders the loss of pulp inevitable (Figure 5.13).

Diagnosis and treatment

A periapical radiograph is essential to assess the state of root development, as this will dictate the type of treatment required. Radiographically, one of the two following situations will be present:

- root development complete;
- root development incomplete.

If the **root development is complete**, obturation with gutta-percha can be carried out. It is useful to remember that trauma to the front teeth is likely to have inflicted some injury to the periodontal ligament. This could lead to some external root resorption. To avoid this, an interim dressing with calcium hydroxide in the root canal should always be carried out and left for a period of at least 3–4 weeks before final obturation of the root canal with gutta-percha.

In cases where **root development is incomplete**, obturation with gutta-percha is not possible as the root canal and the apex can be wide open. The management of non-vital teeth with incomplete root development is discussed below.

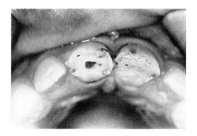

Figure 5.13 Photograph of exposed coronal pulp tissue showing large pulp contamination of tooth 11

Sedation

It may be necessary to use **inhalation sedation** in the management of complicated crown fractures. Children who present with complicated crown fractures have usually suffered a distressing traumatic episode. In addition, many clinicians may be faced with difficulty in obtaining good analgesia in order to carry out the necessary pulp treatment as described in this chapter. This is usually related to the inflamed state of the exposed pulp and also due to a heightened state of anxiety of the child patient. In these cases the role of nitrous oxide inhalation sedation cannot be overemphasized. It helps by:

- reducing the state of anxiety;
- providing relative analgesia and so helps in obtaining total pulpal analgesia, essential for pulp treatment.

ENDODONTIC TREATMENT OF NON-VITAL PERMANENT TEETH WITH INCOMPLETE ROOT DEVELOPMENT

The endodontic management of a non-vital, young permanent tooth can often be complicated, owing to the incomplete root development and a wide-open apex. The open apex makes obturation of the root canal with conventional methods difficult as there is no apical stop against which the root filling can be condensed (Figure 5.14).

In the past, before the introduction of root end closure techniques, a surgical approach was often used to treat such teeth. However, this

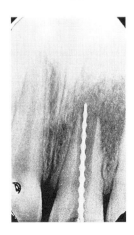

Figure 5.14 Radiograph of traumatized left central incisor with wide open apex

is usually not done for two reasons. First, the thin walls of an immature root canal are prone to fracture either during the preparation of an undercut for the apical amalgam seal or during its closure. Secondly, the poor crown:root ratio is further compromised when root substance is removed during an apicectomy. Therefore, a conservative endodontic approach, aimed at achieving a hard tissue barrier, preferably at the end of the root, against which a gutta percha filling can be condensed, is used in the treatment of such teeth.

In this procedure, known as the **apexification technique**, the root canals are accessed, mechanically cleansed and filled with a medicament, which then stimulates the formation of a hard tissue barrier in young permanent teeth with incomplete root development. Calcium hydroxide is the most widely used root canal medicament and is the mainstay of the apexification technique (Figure 5.15).

Role of calcium hydroxide in apexification

Clinical and experimental studies have shown that when calcium hydroxide is used in the root canal, the healing of the peri-radicular tissues, including the arrest of any inflammatory resorption, and the formation of an apical hard tissue barrier, occurs with a high rate of predictability. It has been shown that 90% of non-vital teeth treated with calcium hydroxide show evidence of healing periapical bony lesions. The use of calcium hydroxide is therefore recommended in the endodontic treatment of young permanent teeth with persistent chronic infection and those with large apical areas. At the same time, it must be emphasized that there **must be a complete coronal seal** so that bacterial reinfection of the root canal does not occur between visits.

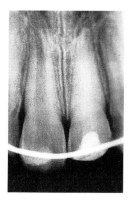

Figure 5.15 Radiograph showing root canal of tooth 21 dressed with calcium hydroxide

Calcium hydroxide is used in these situations as a root canal dressing until there is a resolution of the infection or the apical area, following which final obturation with gutta-percha is carried out. An added advantage is that it is also a strong bactericidal agent, though it loses its potency with time. Perhaps the best-known action of calcium hydroxide is its role in the induction of a hard tissue barrier, which forms the basis for the apexification technique. The exact mechanism of the apical hard tissue barrier formation is not known. The barrier consists of a layer of tissue, first coagulated by calcium hydroxide and later calcified by deposition of calcium from the systemic circulation (Figure 5.16).

Success rates in excess of 95% have been reported for the apexification technique. Closure of the apex is achieved more rapidly in children between the ages of 11 and 15 years and in cases with apices 2 mm or less in diameter, owing to the need for less calcific tissue.

The apexification technique

This technique is employed for the endodontic management of non-vital young permanent teeth with incomplete root development. The clinical procedure is as follows:

- **Gain access** to the root canal and first establish a working length, avoiding any trauma to the apical barrier at subsequent visits when the root canal is re-accessed.

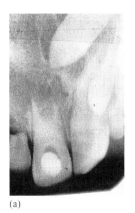

(a)

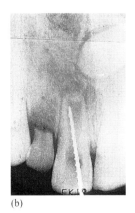

(b)

Figure 5.16 Treatment of open apex: (a) radiograph showing wide-open apex; (b) radiograph taken 18 months later showing formation of a hard tissue barrier

- **Debride** the root canal thoroughly, but carefully, with Hedstrom files and irrigate, as the walls of an immature root canal are usually thin and the root prone to fracture.
- **Dry** the root canal with paper points.
- **Spin calcium hydroxide** into the root canal with a Lentulo spiral filler and compress it lightly towards the apex with a cotton pledget to ensure contact with vital tissue.
- A **dry pledget of cotton wool** is placed in the pulp chamber and access cavity filled with a glass ionomer cement, preventing any coronal leakage.
- A **periapical radiograph** may then be taken to ensure that the root canals are adequately filled with calcium hydroxide.

Many calcium hydroxide preparations are commercially available (Hypocal[R], Pulpdent[R], Rootcal[R]). Their main advantage is that they are radio-opaque and can easily be seen on radiographs. Alternatively, pure grade calcium hydroxide powder, mixed in a ratio of 7 : 1 with barium sulphate for radio-opacity, can be used. This should be mixed with distilled water, saline or propylene glycol, to a paste of required consistency.

Follow-up

The patient is usually reviewed after three or four months for radiographic review and for replacement of calcium hydroxide in the root canal. At each of the follow-up visits:

- Take a periapical X-ray to check for periapical healing and the formation of the hard tissue barrier (Figure 5.16b).
- Re-access the root canal and irrigate with 1% hypochlorite solution to remove the old calcium hydroxide from the root canal.
- Check clinically by introducing a gutta-percha point into the root canal and tapping it gently to feel for an 'apical stop'.

Generally, a file should not be used to check for an **apical stop** because of the risk of perforating the apical barrier, which can be fragile in its early stages of formation. From the time an apical stop is first detected, usually up to 12–18 months after the initial treatment, the root canal is dressed with calcium hydroxide for a further period of 3 months. This is in order to reinforce the apical barrier, after which permanent obturation of the root canal with gutta-percha can be performed.

The hard tissue barrier should be located as apical as possible, ideally around the apex of the tooth. It is useful to remember that it is the level at which calcium hydroxide meets vital tissue capable of hard tissue formation that determines the position of the barrier. To avoid a hard tissue barrier forming inside the root canal, for example somewhere in the apical third, the operator should ensure that the entire length of the root canal is filled with calcium hydroxide.

In teeth with incomplete root development where there is a wide-open apex, granulation tissue can grow into the root canal, especially if there is insufficient calcium hydroxide in the canal. If this happens, a calcific barrier is formed at the point of contact between the vital granulation tissue and calcium hydroxide. This can result in a barrier being formed anywhere in the root canal (Figure 5.17). A good periapical radiograph to determine the working length is therefore necessary at the start of the apexification procedure.

Obturation with gutta-percha

Even though a hard tissue barrier is formed, usually quite predictably, with the use of the apexification technique, the root canals are usually still wide (Figure 5.16b), making the final obturation difficult. Depending on the size of the lumen of the root canal the thickest gutta-percha that can easily be passed as far as the apical barrier should be selected. Sometimes, in cases where the root canal is too wide, two or more thick gutta-percha points can be rolled together on a warm glass slab and used as the master point. The tip of the customized gutta-percha point is then warmed by passing it once through a flame, and introduced immediately into the root canal, pressing steadily, but not too hard, against the apical barrier. Accessory points are then used as necessary.

Alternatively, thermoplasticized gutta-percha can be used. This technique involves injecting molten gutta-percha into the root canal system. The *Obtura II system* (QED, Peterborough, UK) is available which heats a high molecular weight gutta-percha to a temperature of

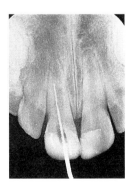

Figure 5.17 Radiographs showing the formation of a dentine barrier in a root canal related to the ingress of granulation tissue

about 160–200°C, which can then be extruded directly into the root canals with a cannula (Figure 5.18a). An effective obturation of root canals with wide lumens is possible with the use of this technique (Figure 5.18b,c).

Apexogenesis versus apexification

Wherever possible, efforts should be made to preserve the vitality of the radicular pulp by carrying out conservative techniques, such as pulp capping, partial pulpotomy and coronal pulpotomy. By maintaining the vitality of the radicular pulp, root development and apical

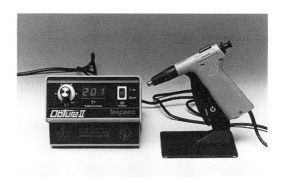

(a)

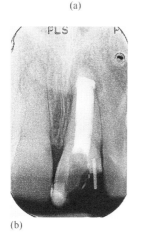

(b)

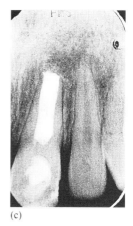

(c)

Figure 5.18 Root canal filling with plasticized gutta-percha: (a) the Obtura II system; (b) root canal filled with gutta-percha using Obtura; (c) follow-up radiograph showing completely sealed root canal

closure by normal cellular mechanisms (**apexogenesis**) is ensured. Only when the pulp vitality cannot be preserved, in spite of best efforts, should the pulp be extirpated and artificial means used to gain a hard tissue barrier (**apexification**).

One of the main drawbacks of the apexification technique is that it does not induce any qualitative increase in the root dimensions. Because of the loss of vitality there will be no further deposition of dentine or cementum. All that can be achieved is apexification, and a hard tissue barrier against which a root filling can be condensed. This can pose a problem where loss of vitality occurs at a very young age with a grossly underdeveloped root. In such cases, even though a hard tissue barrier can be induced and root canals obturated with gutta-percha, the root remains inherently weak and therefore prone to root fracture if any further trauma occurs.

It should thus be remembered that the apexification technique, useful as it might be for the treatment of non-vital young permanent teeth, should only be used when the more conservative efforts aimed at maintaining the vitality of the radicular pulp have failed.

SUMMARY

The management of traumatized young permanent incisors with exposed pulps and incomplete root development is challenging. The preservation of pulp vitality to allow root development is essential. Treatment with calcium hydroxide for apexification when vitality cannot be maintained will usually result in a favourable outcome for most teeth with complicated crown fractures.

REFERENCES AND FURTHER READING

Andreasen, J.O. and Andreasen, F.M. (1994) *Textbook and Colour Atlas of Traumatic Injuries to the Teeth*, 3rd edn. Munksgaard, Copenhagen

Chawla, H.S. (1986) Apical closure in non-vital young permanent teeth using one calcium hydroxide dressing. *Journal of Dentistry for Children*, **53**, 44–47

Cvek, M. (1978) A clinical report on a partial pulpotomy with a capping with calcium hydroxide in permanent incisors with complicated crown fractures. *Journal of Endodontics*, **4**, 232–237

Fuks, A., Chosak, A. and Edelman, E. (1987) Partial pulpotomy as an alternative for exposed pulps in crown fractured permanent incisors. *Endodontics and Dental Traumatology*, **3**, 100–102

Ghose, L.J., Baghdady, V.S. and Hikmat, B.Y. (1987) Apexification of immature apices of pulpless permanent anterior teeth with calcium hydroxide. *Journal of Endodontics*, **13**, 285–290

Mackie, I.C. and Worthington, H.V. (1988) The closure of open apices in non-vital immature incisor teeth. *British Dental Journal*, **165**, 169–174

Tronstad, L., Andreasen, J.O., Hasselgren, G., Kristerson, L. and Riis. I. (1981) pH changes in dental tissues after root canal filling with calcium hydroxide. *Journal of Endodontics*, **7**, 17–21

Chapter 6

Displacement injuries: luxation, avulsion, intrusion, concussion and other displacement injuries

M.S. Duggal

From an anatomical, therapeutic and prognostic point of view, at least six different types of luxation injuries can be identified:

- concussion;
- subluxation;
- lateral luxation;
- intrusive luxation;
- extrusive luxation;
- exarticulation or avulsion.

All are dealt with in this chapter, with the exception of avulsions which are discussed in Chapter 7.

CONCUSSION AND SUBLUXATION

Aetiology

Concussion results from a jarring impact on the tooth, usually in the axial direction. Patients can complain of acute pain on biting for a few days, as a result of bleeding and oedema of the periodontal ligament. When a greater impact results in slight loosening of the tooth without displacement from the socket, it is referred to as *subluxation*.

Diagnosis and clinical recognition

Diagnosis involves both thorough clinical and radiographic examination. In these patients there may well be several different injuries present at the same time. Thus it would not be unusual for one incisor to be luxated while another has sustained an enamel–dentine fracture (see Figure 6.3). All teeth present must be systematically examined and checked for displacements. In many cases this examination may be painful and cause distress, particularly in a young child. It is sometimes useful to use some form of sedation, for which inhalation sedation is ideal.

Alternatively it may be necessary to place some local analgesia and wait until the tissues have become anaesthetized before carrying out an assessment of tooth displacements. Because in most cases of displacement local analgesia is required anyway, the early injection does not mean unnecessary treatment.

Clinical signs and symptoms

- Pain on exerting slight digital pressure on the teeth.
- Percussion is very painful and so should not be carried out.
- In cases of subluxation, there might be traces of bleeding in the sulcus due to damage to the gingival fibres.

Displacement injuries such as concussions and subluxations require immediate treatment to ensure a good prognosis.

Radiographic examination

Radiographs must be taken of each traumatized tooth:

- Appropriate radiographs, usually periapical views, should be taken.
- All teeth suspected of sustaining damage must be radiographed.
- In most cases, separate views taken at different angulations (15 degrees).

Sensibility tests should be carried out to assess pulp vitality

Sensibility testing, especially in very young children, at the time of injury is usually of no diagnostic value as an erratic or exaggerated response will be obtained.

Subluxated teeth may be either concussed or the periapical tissues damaged or torn. In these cases the sensibility test(s) may well be negative, but they are important in order to monitor recovery of the tooth.

Clinical treatment and follow-up

- Electric pulp testing and testing for thermal stimuli with ethyl chloride should be performed 4 weeks after the injury.
- Periapical radiographs, 4-monthly in the first year and 6-monthly in the second year to assess continuous root growth and any periapical pathology.

There is only a slight risk of concussed or subluxated teeth becoming non-vital, but a thorough follow-up is essential (Figure 6.1). Teeth with incomplete root development and an open apex are more likely to remain vital.

LATERAL LUXATION

A lateral luxation is usually as a result of a horizontal force that displaces the tooth either labially or palatally (Figure 6.2). The displacement of the tooth invariably involves the fracture of the alveolar socket walls.

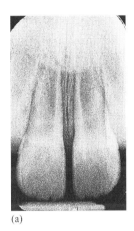
(a)

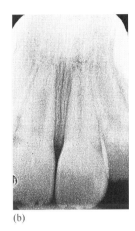
(b)

Figure 6.1 Serial radiographs taken to follow up an injury to maxillary permanent central incisor: (a) following subluxation; (b) 12 months after the injury, showing continued root development

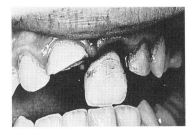

Figure 6.2 Photograph of lateral luxation of a central incisor (21), and complicated fracture of 11

Diagnosis and clinical recognition

In diagnosing luxation of teeth, it is important to test each tooth carefully with the finger tips for mobility and any possible displacement. Even a minor displacement of a tooth can lead to rupture of the apical vessels and compromise the tooth's vitality. As most cases of trauma to the anterior teeth involve young children, the affected teeth may often be inherently crooked and displaced. If a child is in the 'ugly duckling' stage of tooth eruption and development displacement of teeth may be difficult to diagnose.

As part of the clinical diagnosis it is important to question both child and parent as to whether the teeth have been moved or whether the position of the teeth at diagnosis is the norm. Sometimes it is a good idea to ask parents if the teeth are in the same place as usual or even to ask to see recent school photograph(s).

When diagnosing luxated teeth:

- the traumatized teeth usually appear obviously displaced;
- if displaced palatally a luxated tooth can result in interference in occlusion on closing the teeth together (Figure 6.2);
- there may be bleeding evident from the marginal gingivae;
- the tooth may be mobile, but in many cases it may feel firm.

Radiographic examination is essential

As with all cases of trauma involving the teeth, good high-contrast radiographs are essential. A dental practitioner should never be tempted not to take a radiograph of a traumatized tooth, even if he or she thinks the damage is minor. As discussed in Chapter 3, the increasing extent of litigation means that adequate records must be kept of all dental trauma. This includes appropriate radiographs.

In cases of luxation, radiographs are important because:

- it is important to rule out root fracture before any treatment is carried out;
- two periapical radiographs with differing tube angulation or a periapical and an occlusal radiograph should be taken, as one radiograph may not detect a root fracture;
- they are also required to assess the state of root development.

Treatment

There are two treatment principles for the immediate treatment of luxation injuries:

- reduction;
- immobilization.

Reduction

- **Reposition mobile teeth with gentle finger pressure**. This is usually possible in most patients who seek treatment within 12 hours of the tooth being displaced. In the case of upper incisors, both labial and palatal local analgesia is required before the teeth are repositioned, and for lower incisors an inferior dental nerve block should be administered. Sedation, in the form of inhalation sedation (relative analgesia) may also be helpful.
- **In those cases where it is not possible to reposition displaced teeth** with gentle digital pressure, especially in patients who do not seek immediate treatment, they should be left alone.

Teeth should *never* be repositioned forcibly or surgically. Evidence suggests that this can lead to further trauma to the periodontal ligament and could produce ankylosis and root resorption. In such cases, healing should be allowed to occur, usually for about two weeks and then the teeth repositioned using a simple upper removable appliance (Figure 6.3).

Immobilization

Non-rigid 'physiological' splinting should be applied for a period of no more than two weeks. The various splinting methods are discussed

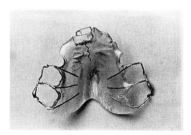 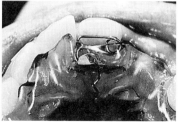

Figure 6.3 Repositioning a luxated incisor: (a) upper removable appliance used to reposition a luxated left central maxillary incisor; (b) appliance in place

in Chapter 11. A thin orthodontic wire, no more than 0.3 mm in diameter, bonded to the teeth with composite resin, is the method of choice (Figure 6.4).

Follow-up

Teeth with incomplete root development

Pulp healing is usually excellent and over 90% of luxated teeth with incomplete root development or open apices will retain vitality. The follow-up and endodontic implications for luxated teeth depend on the state of root development. The steps to be taken are:

- **Sensibility testing** with an electric pulp tester should be **every two months** in the first year. The results of the tests should be interpreted with great caution. It is important to remember that there may be no response to sensibility testing until a few months after the trauma. However, endodontic treatment must not be undertaken unless other clinical signs and symptoms or radiographic evidence might suggest that the pulp is necrotic.
- **Radiographic assessment** should be made on a 3-monthly basis for the first year and 6-monthly in the second year. Look for the following sequelae:

  - continuous root development, as a definite sign that the pulp is vital;
  - apical pathology or inflammatory root resorption, if present: root canal is accessed, mechanically cleaned and filled with non-hard

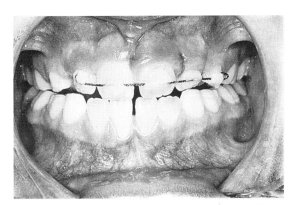

Figure 6.4 Physiological light wire splint placed on maxillary incisors to stabilize luxated and repositioned teeth

setting calcium hydroxide (e.g. Hypocal®): calcium hydroxide is replaced every 3–4 months until resorption has been arrested or a hard tissue barrier achieved before the root canal is obturated with gutta-percha;

– pulp canal obliteration, when no intervention is required, as this usually means the tooth is vital. The arguments against carrying out an elective endodontic treatment have been presented in Chapter 5.

Teeth with complete root development and closed apex

A very high proportion, some two-thirds, of luxated teeth with closed apices will become non-vital. Diagnosis is made from sensibility tests completed over a period of time, clinical signs and symptoms and periodic radiographs. Calcium hydroxide should always be used as an interim dressing before obturating the root canal with gutta-percha. This reduces the risk of inflammatory resorption.

INTRUSIVE LUXATIONS

Intrusive luxations, or intrusions, result from an axial force applied to the incisal edge of the tooth that results in the tooth being driven into the socket (Figure 6.5a).

Sequelae of intrusion

The sequelae of intrusion are either:

- loss of vitality; or
- ankylosis and replacement root resorption.

Loss of pulp vitality

This type of injury results in severe damage to both the pulp and the periodontal ligament. Invariably, all intruded teeth that have closed apices lose the pulp vitality. Teeth where the root development is incomplete, or where the apex is still open, have a 50% chance of retaining pulp vitality.

Loss of pulp vitality also means that inflammatory root resorption may develop unless timely endodontic intervention is carried out (Figure 6.5b).

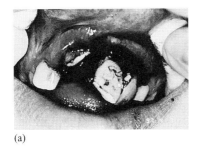

(a)

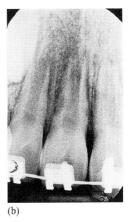

(b)

Figure 6.5 Examples of intruded teeth: (a) intruded right maxillary central incisor; (b) extensive external root resorption involvement of teeth 11 and 21 after loss of vitality following intrusion

Ankylosis and replacement root resorption

Severe injury to the periodontal ligament means that ankylosis followed by replacement resorption may develop. Teeth where root development is complete are more at risk from this complication, compared with teeth with open apices.

Management of intruded teeth

The treatment strategy depends upon the state of root development. Therefore, a periapical radiograph to assess the state of root development is required at the first visit.

Teeth with incomplete root development and open apices

Spontaneous re-eruption over a period of a few weeks can be expected and teeth should be monitored for vitality. These teeth can therefore be left alone and monitored over the following months.

Follow-up protocol

As over half such teeth will become non-vital, constant monitoring of the state of the pulp is required with:

- pulp sensibility testing ever 4 weeks in the first year;
- radiographic assessment after 4 weeks, 8 weeks and then 3-monthly, to monitor apical area, continuous root growth and any root resorption.

At the first sign or symptom of pulp death, such as pain, abscess or inflammatory resorption *at the apical area*, the root canal is accessed, necrotic pulp extirpated and the root canal filled with calcium hydroxide. Treatment with calcium hydroxide is continued until there is evidence that there is no further resorption or of a hard tissue barrier. Gutta-percha is then used to obturate the root canal (see also Chapter 5).

If spontaneous re-eruption does not occur over the ensuing 3–4 months following intrusion, orthodontic extrusion is undertaken as described later in this chapter.

Teeth with complete root development

It is unusual for such teeth to re-erupt spontaneously and therefore they will require orthodontic extrusion. Also, it should be presumed that all intruded teeth with closed apices will become non-vital and would therefore require endodontic management.

Orthodontic extrusion of intruded teeth

Owing to the risk of developing ankylosis and external resorption, orthodontic extrusion should be undertaken within 2–3 weeks following the trauma.

In the authors' experience, most intruded teeth can be managed with simple **removable appliances**. A bracket is attached to the intruded tooth and an upper removable appliance, with Adams' cribs and a whip spring, is constructed to engage the bracket (Figure 6.6). The long arm of the whip spring is activated incisally and is usually effective in extruding the tooth in 3–4 weeks. In some cases of severe intrusion, where very little tooth is actually visible, gingival surgery may be required to expose a small area of the crown to which a bracket can be attached.

In a small number of cases, a **fixed appliance** may be required to extrude an intruded tooth orthodontically. The unaffected maxillary teeth are bracketed and an arch wire fitted. A bracket is then fixed to the intruded tooth which is attached by elastics or springs to the arch wire. Placed under tension, the appliance slowly extrudes the affected tooth (Figure 6.7).

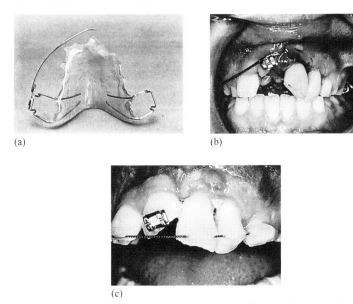

(a)   (b)

(c)

Figure 6.6 Photographs showing an upper removal appliance with whip spring to extrude a tooth: (a) appliance design; (b) appliance in the mouth with spring activated; (c) extrusion of tooth successfully completed in 6 weeks

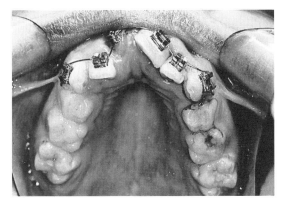

Figure 6.7 Photograph of intruded tooth 11 being extruded with fixed orthodontics

Orthodontic extrusion versus surgical repositioning

It is generally believed that the surgical repositioning of intruded teeth increases the risk of ankylosis and external root resorption (Turley *et al.*, 1987). There is certainly some evidence to support this view, but further research needs to be carried out before ruling out surgical repositioning as a treatment option. It is our view, at the present time, that orthodontic extrusion should be the preferred method of treating intruded teeth.

Endodontic implications

For all intruded teeth with closed apices, the root canal treatment should be initiated as soon as orthodontic extrusion exposes the cingulum area and allows an access cavity to be made. Calcium hydroxide should be used as an interim root canal dressing material and replaced every 3–4 months until there is clear radiographic evidence that root resorption has not occurred or has arrested. Final obturation with gutta-percha is then achieved (see Chapter 5).

EXTRUSIVE LUXATIONS

With extrusive luxations, or extrusions, the tooth appears to be partially displaced axially out of the socket.

Clinical examination

The following may be revealed by clinical exmination:

- the tooth may appear elongated;
- the tooth may also feel quite loose;
- there may be associated bleeding from the periodontal ligament.

Radiographic examination usually shows an increase in periodontal ligament space.

Immediate management

- Reposition the tooth with digital pressure, using local analgesia if necessary.
- Splint for 2–3 weeks using a 'physiological' splint (see Chapter 11).

Sometimes, if the child is particularly upset, some form of sedation may be required. Usually, as the treatment is needed immediately, relative analgesia (inhalation sedation) will be the method of choice.

Follow-up and management of complications

Loss of vitality is common and should be monitored both clinically and radiographically. Teeth with open apices do better than teeth with closed apices, where some 50% may lose pulp vitality. In teeth where pulp necrosis is diagnosed, endodontic treatment is carried out with calcium hydroxide being used as an interim root canal dressing material.

External root resorption, usually the inflammatory type, is managed with calcium hydroxide used in the root canal as a long-term medicament, and replaced every 3–4 months until there is radiographic evidence of its arrest.

SUMMARY

Most luxated teeth can effectively be managed by the simple principles of repositioning, splinting, careful monitoring of pulp vitality and timely endodontic treatment if or when loss of vitality occurs. The use of calcium hydroxide as a root canal dressing material reduces the chance of root resorption occurring. Complacency in the critical areas of clinical and radiographic monitoring can be disastrous, with root resorption an unfortunately common cause of failure.

REFERENCES AND FURTHER READING

Andreasen, F.M. (1986) Transient apical breakdown and its relationship to colour and sensibility changes after luxation injuries to teeth. *Endodontics and Dental Traumatology*, **2**, 9–19

Andreasen, J.O. (1970) Etiology and pathogenesis of traumatic injuries. A clinical study of 1,298 cases. *Scandinavian Journal of Dental Research*, **78**, 329–342

Andreasen, F.M. and Andreasen, J.O. (1987) Occurrence of pulp canal obliteration after luxation injuries in the permanent dentition. *Endodontics and Dental Traumatology*, **3**, 103–115

Andreasen, J.O. and Andreasen, F.M. (1994) *Textbook and Colour Atlas of Traumatic Injuries to the Teeth*, 3rd edn. Munksgaard, Copenhagen

Awang, H., Hill, F.J. and Davies, E.H. (1985) An investigation of three polymeric materials for acid etch splint reconstruction. *Journal of Paediatric Dentistry*, **1**, 55–60

Crona-Larson, G. and Noren, J.G. (1989) Luxation injuries to permanent teeth – a retrospective study of etiological factors. *Endodontics and Dental Traumatology*, **13**, 230–238

Kinirons, M.J. and Sutcliffe, P.J. (1991) Traumatically intruded permanent incisors: a study of treatment and outcome. *British Dental Journal*, **170**, 144–146

Kisterson, L. and Andreasen, J.O. (1983) The effect of splinting upon periodontal and pulpal healing after auto-transplantation of mature and immature permanent incisors in monkeys. *International Journal of Oral Surgery*, **12**, 239–249

Mackie, I.C. (1992) An investigation of replantation of traumatically avulsed permanent incisor teeth. *British Dental Journal*, **172**, 17–20

Mandel, U. and Vidik, A. (1989) Effect of splinting on the mechanical and histological properties of the healing periodontal ligament in the vervet monkey. *Archives of Oral Biology*, **34**, 209–217

Miyashin, M., Ishikawa, M. and Hasimoto, Y. (1986) Tissue reactions after experimental luxation injuries in immature rat teeth. *Endodontics and Dental Traumatology*, **2**, 196–204

Rock, W.P. and Grundy, M.C. (1981) The effect of luxation and subluxation upon the prognosis of traumatised teeth. *Journal of Dentistry*, **9**, 224–230

Turley, P.K., Crawford, L.B. and Carrington, K.W. (1987) Traumatically intruded teeth. *Angle Orthodontist*, **57**, 234–244

Turley, P.K., Joiner, M.W. and Hellstrom, S. (1989) The effect of orthodontic extrusion on traumatically intruded teeth. *American Journal of Orthodontics*, **85**, 47–56

Chapter 7
Displacement injuries: avulsions

M.S. Duggal

Avulsion (exarticulation) of the permanent teeth can occur at any age, but is most common in young permanent dentitions because of the incomplete root development and the resilience of the periodontal ligament. However, sporting injuries can lead to teeth being avulsed at any age. It is usually a horizontal impact that results in the exarticulation of teeth from the socket.

The management of avulsed teeth has evolved slowly over the past 20 years. Most treatment methods are aimed at preventing either inflammatory resorption, or ankylosis followed by replacement resorption. However, due to a large number of prognostic factors influencing the long-term success, tooth loss following reimplantation is a frustrating but a frequent outcome. In recent years, based on extensive research a variety of measures have been suggested which aim to optimize the healing of the periodontal ligament and improve the prognosis of replanted teeth. It is the authors' view that a protocol for the replantation of avulsed teeth and its rationale is not widely understood by dental practitioners. In this chapter the management of avulsed teeth is dealt with, first by describing the techniques used and secondly by answering a series of questions which are commonly asked.

RATIONALE OF TREATMENT

- **Reimplantation** should be accomplished as soon as possible.
- **Radiographs** are needed after reimplantation to ensure that the avulsed tooth is properly back in its socket.
- **Splinting** with a physiological splint is needed for 8–10 days.
- **Root canal** treatment to remove necrotic tissue is usually required and should be instituted as soon as possible.
- **Follow-up** appointments are needed at frequent intervals until the tooth is stabilized, symptom free, the root canal treatment has been completed and to monitor any root resorption.
- **Long-term** follow-up is required.

DIAGNOSIS AND CONSIDERATIONS FOR TREATMENT PLANNING

When a patient presents with an avulsed tooth or teeth, the following factors should be considered before the approach to treatment is made. The most important factor with avulsed teeth is the time that the tooth or teeth have been out of the mouth. There has been considerable research on this subject (Andreasen and Andreasen, 1994), indicating that this one factor is critical to prognosis.

The following factors governing treatment approaches should be considered:

Clinical

- Time of **accident**.
- **Time elapsed** since accident.
- **Storage medium**, if any, of avulsed tooth.
- Possible bacterial **contamination** of root surfaces with dirt or debris.
- Possible **damage** to root surfaces.
- Stage of **root development** – open or closed apices.
- **Cooperation** of patient.
- **Soft tissue** damage, oedema or lacerations.

Radiographic

Radiographs should be taken as soon as possible and according to the patient' degree of cooperation. These are required to assess if there is any damage to the other teeth and also to see if there is any damage to the alveolar bone. In addition, radiographs are needed to monitor the stage of root development. Often in cases of avulsion the tooth has been wrenched from the socket in an outward and upward or downward motion. In doing this the tooth damages the alveolar bone, causing fractures (Figure 7.1).

It is essential to determine if the aveolar bone cortical plate has been displaced, as it may well affect the ease with which the avulsed tooth can be replaced. In many cases the alveolar bone has to be repositioned first before reimplanting the tooth or teeth. This situation can only be determined by adequate radiographs.

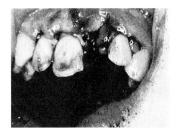

Figure 7.1 Photograph showing severe damage to the alveolar bone associated with an avulsed tooth

TREATMENT METHODS FOR AVULSED TEETH

The step-by-step procedure for reimplanting an avulsed tooth or teeth, in a patient with little or minimal soft tissue swellings, is as follows:

- **Place avulsed tooth**, as soon as patient arrives, **in suitable storage medium**, which can be milk or isotonic solution (Ringer's) if available.
- Take full **history**.
- Check **medical history**.
- Place **local analgesia**.
- Take **radiographs**.
- **Debride** affected soft tissues and gingivae.
- **Reimplant** tooth/teeth when full local analgesia has been obtained.
- **Reposition** tooth/teeth as accurately as possible.
- **Splint** teeth.

Home care

The patient and/or parents will need to be advised as to the home care of the splinted reimplanted tooth/teeth. This advice should cover the following points:

- Clean the splint, soft tissues and teeth several times a day with warm water using a cotton bud or Q-tip[R]. As the patient might find it painful to brush the affected area, Corsydyl[R] (chlorhexidine) mouth rinse should be advised.
- A warm salt-water mouthwash should be recommended starting on the day after the accident. To do this, a glass of water, as warm as can be tolerated, should be taken and a small teaspoon of salt added. The patient should take a mouthful and hold the warm solution under the lip around the affected teeth. This should be repeated until the glass is empty. If carried out several times a day, this will aid healing and give relief from any discomfort.

Analgesics and antibiotics should be prescribed as needed. Antibiotics are often required because in most cases of avulsions the wounds are contaminated with dirt, etc. There is often swelling and tissue damage. The antibiotics of choice are those usually prescribed for dental infections and the latest recommendations should be consulted.

Follow-up visits

First follow-up

The patient should be seen again in 48 hours for the first follow-up visit, at which the following procedure is needed:

- **Check for** mobility, pain, discomfort, swelling.
- **Clean teeth** and splint.
- Clean teeth gently to ensure splint is free of **debris**.

At this stage it may be possible to start the endodontic treatment of the reimplanted tooth/teeth. This is not always the case, but root canal treatment should be started before removing the splint. If the condition of the reimplanted tooth merits the start of endodontics, the procedure is as follows:

- Fit a **rubber dam**.
- Open all reimplanted teeth and **gain access**.
- **Extirpate** all pulp remnants.
- **Debride root canal** with Hedstrom files.
- **Irrigate canal(s)** with saline – multiple washings.
- **Dry canal(s)** with paper points.
- Leave canal(s) **dry**.
- Take **radiograph** to assess working length.
- **Seal access cavity** with glass ionomer cement and make sure the seal is very good.

Second follow-up

The patient will need to be seen again at 8–10 days post trauma, for the second follow-up visit. At this visit the following procedure is needed:

- **Check for** pain, discomfort, swelling.
- Take **radiographs**.
- **Remove** splint.
- Check for excessive **mobility**.

If endodontics has not already been started, and is indicated, it should now be commenced as described above under 'First follow-up' visit.

If the tooth/teeth are reasonably firm and there is/are no other symptoms the patient can be discharged for that visit. However, the tooth/teeth may demonstrate considerable mobility and therefore the patient should be warned to be careful with eating, etc.

Third follow-up

At this visit, approximately 2–3 weeks after the trauma, the following procedure is carried out:

- **Check for** pain, discomfort, swelling.
- Check for excessive **mobility**.
- Fit **rubber dam**.
- Open all reimplanted teeth and **gain access**.
- **Debride root canal** with Hedstrom files.
- Take **diagnostic radiograph**.
- **Irrigate canal(s)** with saline – multiple washings.
- **Dry canal(s)** with paper points.
- Fill root canal with **calcium hydroxide** (Figure 7.2).
- **Reseal** access cavity with glass ionomer cement.

At this point in the treatment, if the tooth/teeth is/are completely symptomless and there is no radiographic evidence of any pathology, such as external or internal resorption, etc., an appointment can be

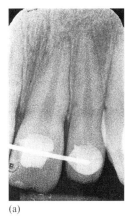

(a)

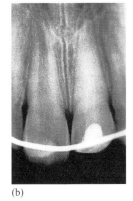

(b)

Figure 7.2 Radiograph of reimplanted tooth: (a) initial radiograph at time of reimplantation; (b) root canal filled with Hypocal^R before removal of the splint

made to carry out a final root canal filling. If the apices of the affected tooth/teeth are open, the usual procedures to achieve a hard tissue barrier are carried out (see Chapter 6).

Some authors prefer to treat the tooth/teeth with calcium hydroxide for at least 9–12 months before the final root canal filling is placed. It is the authors' experience that, given the high risk of root resorption, the final working length is likely to change in the first 12 months. The final root canal filling should therefore be deferred until any resorption has stabilized, to ensure a good obturation of the root canal.

Avulsed teeth with open apices

Children who avulse teeth may often be quite young and the maxillary incisors may have very wide-open apices. If these teeth can be reimplanted very quickly, within minutes, there is a good chance that the pulp tissues may revascularize and even obtain a new innervation. Usually, unfortunately, these teeth are not quickly reimplanted and the chance of revascularization decreases with increasing extra-alveolar time.

COMMON QUESTIONS CONCERNING AVULSED TEETH

Over the years the authors have dealt with many cases of trauma to the teeth, in particular avulsed teeth. Avulsed teeth seem to pose the greatest problems to dentists, and during the course of teaching the subject many questions have been asked us. Accordingly, below we have compiled a selection of the most often asked questions and their answers.

What is a good storage medium and is tooth storage important?

It would be most desirable to reimplant avulsed teeth as quickly as possible, but this may not be possible in many cases. It is essential to prevent the tooth from drying to maintain the maximal viability of the periodontal ligament cells that are still attached to the root surface of the avulsed tooth. Dry storage is not desirable, as research has shown that after 60 minutes of dry storage very few periodontal ligament cells remain viable (Andreasen and Andreasen, 1990).

On the other hand, any storage media must have a favourable osmotic balance with the cells of the pulp and periodontal ligament. Milk is by far the best storage medium. It is commonly available and has a near neutral pH (6.5–6.8) and osmolality which is conducive to the long-term survival of cells. Studies have shown favourable success rates of teeth reimplanted after up to 6 hours of storage in milk (Andreasen and Andreasen, 1990).

The storage medium used is therefore of paramount importance and Table 7.1 gives a summary of the relative qualities of the storage media as reviewed in the literature.

Table 7.1 Possible storage media as recommended from research reported in the literature

Medium	Details
Milk	Excellent media owing to its favourable pH and osmolality. Few virulent micro-organisms owing to pasteurization
Saliva	Allows storage for up to 2 hours. Is hypotonic and not a medium of choice. Contamination of root surface with oral micro-organisms can influence prognosis
Tap water	As bad as dry storage, its hypotonicity causing cell lysis

What advice on the management of avulsed teeth should be given on the telephone?

As the extra-alveolar period is one of the most important determinants of success, it is important to reimplant avulsed teeth as soon as possible. If the parent, guardian or the teacher telephones the surgery following an accident resulting in the avulsion of a tooth, the following advice should be given:

- do not touch the root;
- place back in socket if possible, or in milk, saliva or buccal sulcus in that order of preference;
- attend surgery immediately.

Many parents and teachers could and should manage to push the tooth back into the socket and be encouraged to do so. It does not matter if they replant the tooth back to front, that can be corrected before the placement of the splint.

How should the tooth be reimplanted?

When the patient arrives at the surgery a medical history and a history of the injury should be taken. This should be done briskly, so that the reimplantation can be carried out as soon as possible, in order to minimize the extra-alveolar period for the avulsed tooth.

The following procedure is recommended for reimplantation (also described earlier under 'Treatment methods for avulsed teeth):

- **Local analgesia** should be given before reimplantation of the tooth.
- **Do not handle the avulsed tooth by root**, to minimize the risk of further damage to periodontal ligament.
- **Holding the tooth by the crown**, rinse the root with normal saline using an irrigating syringe, ensuring removal of debris and other foreign bodies.
- **Flush the socket** with saline to remove coagulum, as there is evidence that the presence of the coagulum can lead to an increased risk of ankylosis.
- Holding the tooth by the crown, **push it firmly into the socket**, with local analgesia, both buccal and palatal, especially in children.
- It is important to ensure that the tooth is **seated fully into the socket**.
- A **non-rigid splint**, such as that described in Chapter 11, should be applied for no more than 8–10 days.
- **Check occlusion** to make sure there is no interference.
- Take a periapical **radiograph** after reimplanting the tooth.
- Prescribe **antibiotics** and Corsodyl^R mouth rinse.

Oral hygiene instructions should be given. The maintenance of good oral hygiene is essential for the healing of the gingival fibres. The use of systemic antibiotics at the time of reimplantation prevents bacterial invasion of the pulp and subsequent inflammatory root resorption. It also helps prevent any infection which might result from wound contamination.

What is the rationale of non-rigid and short period of splinting?

The period and type of splinting is critical. In avulsed teeth the injury to the periodontal ligament is severe, making them prone to ankylosis. Prolonged rigid fixation causes a high degree of bone ingrowth into the periodontal space, leading to ankylosis and eventually replacement resorption. Minimal, non-rigid splinting allows physiological 'jiggling' movements of the tooth and favours normal healing of the periodontal ligament and reduces the risk of ankylosis. Splinting with a twistflex wire bonded to one tooth on either side of the reimplanted tooth with composite resin should be adequate (see Chapter 11).

It is also important to remember that when the splint is removed after 8–10 days, the tooth is still very mobile. The patient should be reassured that it will become firm over the next few days and instructions given to avoid biting on the loose tooth and generally to be careful not to damage it further.

How soon should the tooth be reimplanted?

When the patient arrives at the surgery a history of the injury should be taken. This should be done briskly, so that the reimplantation can be carried out as soon as possible, in order to minimize the extra-alveolar period for the avulsed tooth.

Do reimplanted teeth always require endodontic treatment?

Appropriate endodontic management of reimplanted teeth is crucial for long-term success. Most reimplanted teeth will require endodontic treatment except those with very immature root development. The guidelines and the principles which govern the endodontic management of reimplanted teeth are as follows:

Teeth with incomplete root development stored in appropriate medium and reimplanted within 30 minutes

In these cases pulp revascularization is a possibility, as discussed above, and such teeth should be monitored radiographically. However, at the first clinical or radiographic sign of periapical pathology or inflammatory root resorption, the root canal is accessed, pulp extirpated and root canal filled with calcium hydroxide. Revascularization rarely occurs, and so the teeth should be monitored regularly as replacement resorption can be fulminating and cause extensive root resorption over a very short period of time.

In the absence of any signs of periapical pathology and root resorption, continuous root growth should be taken as a definite sign of revascularization (Figure 7.3). Pulp testing with either thermal stimuli or electric pulp testing is unreliable.

Teeth with completed root development

Irrespective of the extra-alveolar period or the method of storage, reimplanted teeth with completed root development should be treated endodontically as soon as possible.

When should the pulp be extirpated?

To minimize the risk of bacterial invasion of a non-vital pulp triggering off inflammatory resorption, the pulp should be extirpated as soon as possible after the reimplantation. The only exception to this rule is teeth with incomplete root development that have been reimplanted within 30 minutes, as described above.

As a general rule, root canal treatment should be started just before the splint is removed. This is because reimplanted teeth still

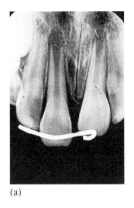
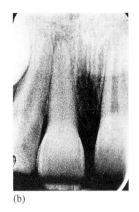

(a)   (b)

Figure 7.3 Radiographs of a reimplanted tooth (11): (a) at time of injury with immature root; (b) at follow-up, showing revascularization and continued root development

demonstrate considerable mobility after the splint removal, gradually becoming firm over a few days. It would therefore be prudent to start the root treatment with the splint still in place to avoid further trauma to the periodontal ligament.

How soon should the root canal be filled and with what?

It has been generally accepted that after extirpation of the pulp the root canals should be filled with a calcium hydroxide paste with water or propylene glycol. Proprietary brands, such as Hypocal^R, offer the additional advantage of being radio-opaque and so can be visualized on periapical film.

Until recently it was recommended that calcium hydroxide be used in the root canals as soon as the pulp was extirpated, usually within 5–7 days of reimplantation. However, there is some concern that use of calcium hydroxide so soon after reimplantation might not be conducive for healing and should be deferred for at least two weeks after the injury. The reason for this is that as at the time of the pulp extirpation the periodontal repair has not been completed, the high pH of calcium hydroxide might cause further inflammation of the already severely traumatized periodontal ligament.

It is therefore recommended that **calcium hydroxide be used two weeks after the reimplantation** so that some repair of the injured periodontal ligament may occur. For the two weeks following extirpation of the pulp, therefore, the root canal should be left unfilled and dry. There is some recent evidence that a medicament, such as Ledermix^R, might be beneficial in this interim period.

If there is any evidence of external root resorption, calcium hydroxide should be used for up to 12 months, being replaced every 3–4 months. However, if there is no evidence of external root resorption in the six months following replantation, the root canal can be obturated with gutta-percha. In teeth with incomplete root development and open apices, calcium hydroxide will need to be used for as long as it takes to develop a hard tissue barrier.

What is the rationale for the use of calcium hydroxide?

Calcium hydroxide has the following properties that make it a long-term root canal medicament of choice in reimplanted teeth:

- The high pH of calcium hydroxide is **bactericidal**.
- It **inhibits inflammatory resorption** by favourably influencing the local environment at resorption sites at the root surface through the dentinal tubules, preventing the dissolution of the mineral component of the tooth by the following possible mechanisms: (a) by necrotizing the cells of the resorption lacunae, and (b) by neutralizing the lactic acid of osteoclasts and macrophages.
- It plays an important role in **hard tissue formation** and repair, as its high pH may stimulate the activity of alkaline phosphatases which in turn promote hard tissue formation.

How frequently are radiographs required?

Periodic periapical radiographs are essential to monitor reimplanted teeth. There is usually no need to take radiographs before the teeth are reimplanted, except where other injuries are suspected, as this only delays reimplantation and increases the extra-alveolar period. The following schedule is suggested:

- immediately after reimplantation if alveolar fracture is suspected;
- after pulp extirpation to estimate the working length;
- after calcium hydroxide filling to ensure adequate filling;
- 1 month later;
- 3-monthly for the first year;
- 4-monthly for the second year;
- yearly thereafter.

If root resorption has not occurred in the first two years it is unlikely to occur. However, yearly radiographic assessment should be made for at least another 3–5 years, perhaps longer, especially in cases where the extra-alveolar period and storage conditions were not favourable.

How is a reimplanted tooth likely to heal?

Once the tooth has been reimplanted it can:

- heal with a normal periodontal ligament;
- heal with ankylosis and undergo replacement resorption;
- undergo inflammatory root resorption.

Healing with a normal periodontal ligament

Only teeth with a short extra-alveolar period and storage in a good medium are likely to demonstrate periodontal healing. Most studies have shown that periodontal healing, with no evidence of any external root resorption, is seen in some 25% of reimplanted teeth (Andreasen, 1995). However, it should be anticipated that two-thirds of reimplanted teeth will show some external root resorption. It is important to understand the resorptive process and its management in order to improve the prognosis of reimplanted teeth.

Healing with ankylosis and replacement resorption

Teeth with a prolonged extra-alveolar period, especially the ones that are not stored in an appropriate medium, are likely to develop ankylosis. Ankylosis is a result of the ingrowth of bone into the periodontal ligament space, until eventually there is a complete bony fusion between the root and the socket walls.

Ankylosis can be diagnosed both clinically and radiographically. Clinically the diagnosis is based upon:

- absence of normal physiological mobility;
- dull, typically metallic, percussion sound;
- infra-occlusion.

Infra-occlusion is pathognomonic of ankylosis in the developing dentition (Figure 7.4).

Radiographic presentation of ankylosis is demonstrated by the lack of a periodontal ligament space (Figure 7.5).

What will eventually happen to ankylosed teeth?

Ankylosed teeth will gradually appear more and more infra-occluded as other teeth grow around them, with the developing alveolar process. In addition, most of the ankylosed teeth will also undergo replacement resorption (Figure 7.5).

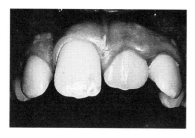

Figure 7.4 Photograph of infra-occluded tooth 21 previously reimplanted

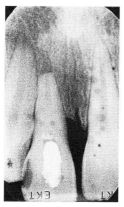

Figure 7.5 Radiograph of an ankylosed reimplanted tooth 11 showing a lack of the periodontal ligament space and replacement resorption

What is replacement resorption?

Bone is a dynamic tissue and is constantly being remodelled by osteoclastic activity to resorb old tissue and by osteoblastic activity to form new bone. Normally, the cementum and the bone are separated by the periodontal ligament, which ensures that the cementum is in no way affected by the constant metabolic activity in the bone. When there is an ankylotic fusion between the cementum and bone the osteoclasts do not differentiate between the cementum and bone, leading to the resorption of the root surface. In addition, the resorbed root is replaced by new bone, hence the term 'replacement resorption'. Radiographically, resorption is evident but there is no periapical area as the resorbed root is being replaced by bony tissue (Figure 7.5).

What should be done once ankylosis and replacement resorption are evident?

Ankylosis and replacement resorption are irreversible and if left to progress lead to a gradual replacement of the periodontal ligament and dentine (Figure 7.6a). Patients are usually concerned about the poor aesthetics associated with infra-occluded teeth and, to a certain extent, composite resin material can be added to the incisal edge of the infra-occluded teeth, to lengthen them to the level of the unaffected adjacent teeth. This usually has to be repeated on subsequent visits, as the other teeth continue to grow relative to the ankylosed tooth.

Usually, ankylosed teeth are not removed, as their surgical removal will entail loss of alveolar bone which would compromise the future placement of implants. In cases of severe infra-occlusion, the following procedure is recommended:

- Withdraw gutta-percha root filling from the tooth.
- De-coronate the tooth and provide patient with an over-denture.
- Leave the root to resorb – it will gradually be replaced with bone.

Such treatment has been shown to preserve the alveolar ridge, making future prosthetic management easier.

What is inflammatory root resorption?

This is a result of mechanical trauma, resulting in the removal of cementoblasts and pre-cementum, and even cementum, from the surface of the root. Microbial stimuli from an infected root canal then provide the necessary impetus for the resorbing cells. If not checked therapeutically, the resorptive process can lead to extensive destruction of the root. Radiographically, inflammatory resorption can be

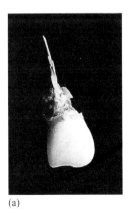

(a)

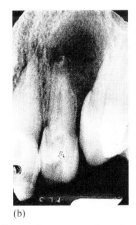

(b)

Figure 7.6 Illustrations of: (a) replacement resorption of the entire root around a gutta-percha root filling; (b) inflammatory resorption of tooth 22

distinguished from replacement resorption, the former presenting with root resorption associated with a periapical area (Figure 7.6b).

How can inflammatory resorption be treated?

As soon as inflammatory resorption is evident radiographically, the root canal should be accessed, necrotic pulp extirpated and root canal filled with calcium hydroxide if the tooth has not already had its pulp extirpated. If inflammatory resorption is seen in a reimplanted tooth that has already had endodontic treatment started, a rigorous regimen of repeated treatments with calcium hydroxide should be started.

Calcium hydroxide, used with frequent changes over 6–9 months, effectively arrests the resorptive process. In this regard, inflammatory resorption differs from replacement resorption as the treatment of the latter remains beyond our therapeutic competence.

What factors influence the prognosis of replanted teeth?

Research has shown that the two most important prognostic factors for replanted teeth are:

- extra-alveolar period;
- type and method of storage medium.

    Other factors that influence the prognosis are:

- stage of root development;
- mechanical damage during exarticulation and reimplantation;
- treatment of socket;
- period and method of splinting;
- endodontic treatment;
- oral hygiene during the period of healing.

The chances of periodontal healing are greatly reduced after 30 minutes of dry storage. However, periodontal healing has been shown to have occurred in teeth that have been reimplanted after storage in a physiological medium, such as milk, for up to 6 hours.

Some clinicians prefer not to reimplant avulsed teeth if they have been out for more than two or three hours, especially if they have been allowed to dry. The authors feel that reimplantation should be carried out even for those teeth that have been avulsed for up to 6 hours, or even longer.

There is no doubt that such teeth will ankylose and undergo replacement resorption; however, in a young child it could have the following advantages:

- resorption takes several years;
- a child can have a natural tooth in place of an upper removable denture;
- replacement resorption will ensure a good bony infill;
- the height of the alveolar ridge is maintained making future prosthesis, such as an implant, easier to place.

LATE REIMPLANTATION

Recently, a few authors have described a technique for reimplanting avulsed permanent teeth with avital periodontal ligaments, resulting from a prolonged extra-alveolar time. The treatment objective in these cases is to achieve ankylosis and is only suitable for use in teenagers and young adults where active growth of the alveolar processes has ceased and infra-occlusion would not be a major problem.

The reimplantation technique is as follows:

- The sockets and soft tissues are allowed to heal for a week.
- The teeth have been stored dry in a refrigerator at 4°C.
- One day prior to reimplantation the root canals of the avulsed teeth are accessed and the necrotic pulps extirpated with barbed broaches.
- The root canals are gently filed and irrigated.
- The teeth are then immersed in a 2.4% sodium fluoride solution (pH 6.5) for 20 minutes.
- The root canals are then obturated with gutta-percha and a zinc oxide–eugenol based sealer.
- The necrotic periodontal ligament is removed with a surgical blade until the root surface is completely clean and there is no soft tissue visible on the surface.
- The root surfaces are then rinsed with saline and teeth left overnight in 3 g amoxycillin made up to 50 ml.

Surgical procedure

A week to 10 days after the trauma, the teeth are surgically replanted, usually under naso-endotracheal anaesthesia. The socket margins are excised and the sockets curetted to remove all blood and granulation tissue (Figure 7.7a). Any periodontal ligament remnants are also removed at the same time, leaving the sockets with clean bony walls.

The avulsed teeth are gently placed in their respective sockets (Figure 7.7b). The labial gingivae are reapplied to the amelocemental junction of the reimplanted teeth using interrupted interdental vertical mattress sutures. A rigid (0.9 mm) round wire is used to splint the teeth with acid etch composite resin (Figure 7.7c). Antibiotics and Corsodyl[R] mouthwash should be prescribed for a period of 7 days postoperatively.

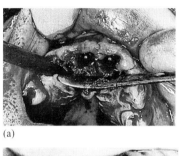

(a)

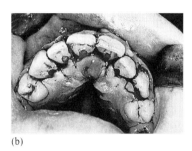

(b)

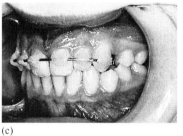

(c)

Figure 7.7 Photographs of technique of late reimplantation of avulsed teeth: (a) socket margins prepared surgically; (b) teeth replaced in sockets; (c) teeth splinted

Follow-up

The splint is left in place for a period of 12 weeks. Postoperative radiographs usually reveal ankylosis of reimplanted teeth at 3 months (Figure 7.8). Radiographic assessment should then be carried out 6-monthly until the tooth/teeth become unsustainable or the patient reaches an age when implants can be considered.

Justification of this technique

In cases where the loss of the viability of the periodontal ligament cells is certain, chemical treatment of the root surface has been advocated (Duggal *et al.*, 1994), the aim being to make the root surface resistant to the resorptive process. Fluoride solutions should be used because of the known effects of the fluoride ion in decreasing the solubility of the dental hard tissues. Also, if the teeth are not replanted, the resulting defect in the alveolar bone in the anterior region would make difficult the provision of an aesthetically

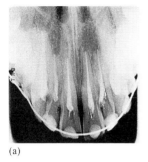
(a)

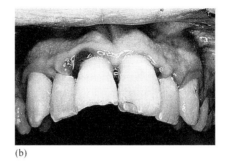
(b)

Figure 7.8 Illustration of a treated case where several teeth were reimplanted after several hours extra-oral: (a) radiograph showing ankylosis; (b) oral appearance of ankylosed teeth

acceptable prosthesis at a later age. There is no doubt that the fluoride treatment will only serve to delay the resorptive process, but with the roots being replaced with bone there will at least be a bony infill in this area, thus restoring the height of the alveolar bone.

Therefore, the technique of avital reimplantation does have a place in the treatment of avulsion injuries. Even though the long-term prognosis of the teeth will be poor, for a few selected cases, it will ensure that the patient reaches the final stages of growth and also maintains the height of the alveolar ridge, thus improving conditions for future restorative management.

SUMMARY

Dental practitioners will occasionally be faced with the task of reimplanting teeth and need to be aware of new developments to maximize the success of the procedure. The successful long-term survival of reimplanted teeth is very satisfying for the dental practitioner and generates goodwill in the community.

REFERENCES AND FURTHER READING

Andersson, L., Bodin, I. and Sorenson, S. (1989) Progression of root resorption following replantation of human teeth after extended extraoral storage. *Endodontics and Dental Traumatology*, **5**, 38–47

Andreasen, J.O. (1975) The effect of splinting upon periodontal healing after replantation of permanent incisors in monkeys. *Acta Odontologica Scandinavica*, **33**, 313–323

Andreasen, J.O. (1981) The effect of pulp extirpation or root canal treatment on periodontal healing after replantation of permanent incisors in monkeys. *Journal of Endodontics*, **7**, 245–251

Andreasen, J.O. (1992) *Atlas of Replantation and Transplantation of Teeth*, 1st edn. Mediglobe SA, Basle

Andreasen, J.O. and Andreasen, F.M. (1990) *Essentials of Traumatic Injuries to the Teeth*, 1st edn. Munskgaard, Copenhagen

Andreasen, J.O. and Andreasen, F.M. (1994) *Textbook and Colour Atlas of Traumatic Injuries to the Teeth*, 3rd edn. Munksgaard, Copenhagen

Andreasen, J.O. (1995) Replantation of 400 avulsed permanent teeth. I. diagnosis of healing complications. *Endodontics and Dental Traumatology*, **11**, 51–58

Blomlof, L. (1981) Milk and saliva as possible storage media for traumatically exarticulated teeth prior to replantation. *Scandinavian Dental Journal*, **8** (suppl.), 1–26

Coccia, C.T. (1980) A clinical investigation of root resorption rates in reimplanted young permanent incisors: a five year study. *Journal of Endodontics*, **6**, 413–420

Duggal, M.S., Toumba, K.J., Russell, J. and Paterson, S. (1994) Replantation of avulsed permanent teeth with avital periodontal ligaments. *Endodontics and Dental Traumatology*, **10**, 282–285

Hammarstrom, L., Blomlof, L., Feiglin, B., Anderson, L. and Lindskog, S. (1986) Replantation of teeth and antibiotic treatment. *Endodontics and Dental Traumatology*, **2**, 51–57

Hammarstrom, L., Blomlof, L. and Lindskog, S. (1989) Dynamics of dentoalveolar ankylosis and associated root resorption. *Endodontics and Dental Traumatology*, **5**, 163–175

Lindskog, S. and Blomlof, L. (1982) Influence of osmolality and composition of storage media on human periodontal ligament cells. *Acta Odontologica Scandinavica*, **40**, 435–441

Malmgren, B., Cvek, M., Lundberg, M. and Frykholm, A. (1984) Surgical treatment of ankylosed and infrapositioned re-implanted permanent incisors in adolescents. *Scandinavian Journal of Dental Research*, **92**, 391–399

Shulman, L.B., Gedalia, I. and Feingold, R.M. (1973) Fluoride concentration in root surfaces and alveolar bone of fluoride-immersed monkey incisors three weeks after replantation. *Journal of Dental Research*, **52**, 1314–1316

Chapter 8

Root fractures

S.A. Fayle

Root fracture is an uncommon injury in both the permanent and primary dentition. The prevalence of root fracture is between 0.5% and 7% of all dental injuries in the permanent dentition (Andreasen and Andreasen, 1994). While these fractures are relatively easy to deal with, many dental practitioners seem to be uneasy about their treatment.

CLASSIFICATION OF ROOT FRACTURE INJURIES

Root fractures may be transverse (horizontal), oblique or vertical. The last type occurs rarely as a primary injury in young permanent incisors, but may result from trauma to a tooth which has already been restored with a post-crown. Posterior teeth, especially those with a large restoration running the length of the tooth (e.g. a mesio-occlusodistal restoration), are also more prone to vertical root fracture.

Transverse and oblique fractures are the most commonly seen type in previously undamaged incisors (Figure 8.1). They may be single or multiple and single horizontal/oblique root fractures carry the best prognosis. The other factor which affects prognosis is the level of the fracture. Horizontal/oblique root fractures may occur at any level of the root. For simplicity, they are usually described according to the third of the root in which they occur: apical third; middle third; coronal third. The more coronal the fracture, the worse the prognosis.

Root fractures occurring near to the cervical level carry the worst prognosis, especially if they communicate with the gingival sulcus or involve part of the crown (crown/root fracture) (Figure 8.2). In these cases, often the only viable approach is to treat the case as a complete decoronation injury. This may be with or without extrusion of the remaining root, although maintenance of the natural crown by permanent rigid splinting to adjacent teeth has been described (Andreasen and Andreasen, 1994).

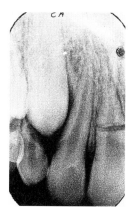

Figure 8.1 Radiograph showing a transverse/oblique root fracture of an incisor

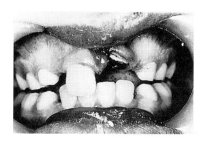

Figure 8.2 Photograph showing decoronated fracture of an incisor

HEALING OF ROOT FRACTURES

Andreasen and Andreasen (1994) have described four modes of healing:

- hard tissue union;
- interposition of fibrous tissue;
- interposition of fibrous tissue and bone;
- interposition of granulation tissue.

Hard tissue union

The fracture is repaired by formation of a dentine-like callus on the pulpal aspect which is followed by ingrowth of cementum-like tissue from the periodontal aspect. This produces a rigid union between the fragments over a period of 2–3 months. This type of healing is probably only possible if the apical and coronal fragments are held in rigid close apposition for a prolonged period.

Interposition of fibrous tissue

Fibrous tissue grows between the fragments, forming a direct communication between the periodontal ligament and the pulp. The radiographic appearance of the periodontal and pulpal edges of the fracture become rounded with time and the coronal fragment is essentially mechanically separate from the apical fragment. This probably occurs in teeth where incomplete reduction of the root fracture has occurred.

Interposition of fibrous tissue and bone

This is essentially similar to interposition of fibrous tissue, but probably occurs in teeth where a reduction of the fracture is even less complete. Radiographically, bone is seen to penetrate along the line of the fracture between the fragments. If the apical fragment maintains its vitality, a lamina dura frequently becomes apparent between this bone and the fracture face.

Interposition of granulation tissue

This does not really constitute normal healing, but signifies frustrated healing, usually secondary to pulpal death in the coronal fragment. Radiographically, the fracture line often becomes more clearly defined, widened, and is usually associated with loss of lamina dura and radiolucency in the alveolar bone adjacent to the fracture line. Clinically, these teeth are often symptomatic, with an increasing tenderness on vertical and lateral pressure as well as pain, swelling and/or sinus formation on the alveolus at the level of the fracture. Such teeth require endodontic intervention (see below).

DIAGNOSIS OF HORIZONTAL/OBLIQUE ROOT FRACTURE

Clinically, a horizontal/oblique root fracture may resemble, and in some cases be clinically indistinguishable from, a luxation or subluxation injury. Occasionally, no clinical injury is apparent, or the tooth involved may have suffered another more obvious injury, e.g. a crown fracture. Where mobility of the coronal fragment is present, the tooth may be perceived to be rotating around a point more coronal than that seen in a normal luxation injury. The tooth is also frequently tender to vertical and horizontal pressure.

Radiographs are required to diagnose a root fracture. For this reason it is essential that periapical radiographs are taken on all teeth thought to have received an injury. Because many root fractures are oblique, teeth where a root fracture is suspected should be radiographed from at least two different angles in the vertical plane. This can usually be accomplished by taking two periapical views, one by bisecting the angle and a second using a paralleling technique. This approach is more likely to identify an oblique fracture which may not be apparent on a single view.

Treatment of horizontal/oblique root fracture (apical and middle third)

Treatment of these types of root fracture is accomplished by:

- **Reduction and repositioning** of the coronal crown/root fragment.
- **Rigid splinting** for 12–14 weeks.
- **Radiographs** taken immediately postoperatively and at 1 and 3 months.
- **Vitality tests** at 1 and 3 months postoperatively.
- **Removal of splint** after 12–14 weeks and mobility checked for.
- Continued **follow-up** at 3-monthly intervals.

The ideal outcome for horizontal/oblique root fracture injuries is healing by hard tissue union. This is thought to be most likely to occur if the fracture is fully reduced and the fracture edges are rigidly held in close apposition for a prolonged period (12–14 weeks).

In practice this is achieved first by reducing any luxation of the coronal fragment by repositioning (usually under local analgesia) and secondly by the placement of a rigid splint, which is left in situ for 12–14 weeks.

A heavy composite and stainless steel wire (0.8–1.0 mm) splint is most appropriate and, if possible, two abutment teeth on either side of the injured tooth/teeth should be included to enhance rigidity. The design and placement of such a splint is described fully in Chapter 11.

Treatment of horizontal/oblique root fracture (coronal third)

Treatment of these types of root fracture is dependent on the location of the fracture line. If the crown is fractured off through the root but close to the gingival margin, the options are:

- dispense with the crown and carry out a root canal treatment with subsequent extrusion and post-crown;
- use crown as a bonded temporary restoration after preliminary root canal with subsequent post-crown;
- rigid splinting of the crown to adjacent teeth after root canal therapy.

These treatments are not easy to accomplish and in most cases are best referred, after emergency care, to a specialist in paediatric or restorative dentistry.

LOSS OF PULPAL VITALITY AND ENDODONTIC INTERVENTION

Between 20% and 44% of root fractured permanent incisors will subsequently lose vitality (Andreasen and Hjorting-Hansen, 1967; Zachrisson and Jacobsen, 1975). The risk of pulpal necrosis is higher in mature teeth and those where significant dislocation of the coronal fragment has occurred. Extrusion, tenderness to percussion, discoloration of the crown, and development of radiolucency in the alveolar bone adjacent to the fracture, may indicate pulpal necrosis. As with other types of injury, a negative result to sensibility testing alone is not necessarily indicative of pulpal necrosis.

If pulpal necrosis does occur, it is usually confined to the coronal fragment, the apical fragment almost always remaining vital (Andreasen and Hjorting-Hansen, 1967). Endodontic intervention should therefore be carried out to the level of the fracture line only, leaving the apical fragment pulp tissue intact. Careful radiographic determination of the working length (to the level of the fracture) is necessary (Figure 8.3a).

Instrumentation and obturation of the canal at this stage can be difficult because of the lack of a mechanical stop, especially in young teeth with wide canals. For this reason, the root canal is usually dressed initially with non-setting calcium hydroxide which encourages the formation of a hard apical barrier, very much in the same way as the apexification technique (see Chapter 6). Final gutta-percha obturation is carried out once a barrier has formed and satisfactory peri-radicular healing has occurred (Figure 8.3b).

PROGNOSIS

Pulpal necrosis occurs in 20–44% of teeth with root fractures. Pulp canal obliteration is also commonly seen, occurring in more than two-

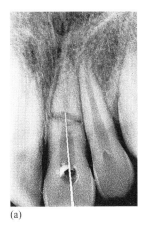
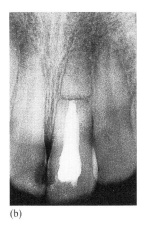

(a)   (b)

Figure 8.3 Treatment of root fractures: (a) diagnostic radiograph to determine working length to the root fracture line; (b) obturation of root canal as far as the fracture

thirds of root fractured permanent incisors (Andreasen *et al.*, 1989). Canal obliteration may occur in either the coronal or radicular fragment, or both. Canal obliteration coronal to the level of the fracture indicates continued vitality of the coronal fragment and only rarely does this lead to pulpal necrosis, although the crown may develop a slightly yellow discoloration.

Root resorption occurs in about 60% of root fractured incisors (Jacobsen and Zachrisson, 1975). *Surface resorption* at the external and internal margins of the fracture, with rounding of the edges, is commonly seen in those teeth healing by interposition of connective tissue. More extensive *external replacement resorption* may also happen. *Tunnelling resorption* on the internal surface of the pulp chamber may also occur, but often resolves spontaneously.

In many cases, these resorptive phenomena are often followed by healing. Conversely, *inflammatory resorption*, which is characterized by bony radiolucency adjacent to the fracture line, indicates pulpal necrosis and endodontic intervention is indicated.

SUMMARY

Root fracture is a relatively uncommon injury. Treatment by repositioning of the coronal fragment and rigid splinting for 12–14 weeks often results in healing of the fracture by hard tissue union or interposition of connective tissue. If pulpal necrosis does occur, it is usually confined to the coronal fragment.

REFERENCES

Andreasen, J.O. and Andreasen, F.M. (1994) *Textbook and Colour Atlas of Traumatic Injuries to the Teeth*, 3rd edn. Munksgaard, Copenhagen

Andreasen, F.M., Andreasen, J.O. and Bayer, T. (1989) Prognosis of root fractured permanent incisors – prediction of healing modalities. *Endodontics and Dental Traumatology*, **5**, 11–22

Andreasen, J.O. and Hjorting-Hansen, E. (1967) Intraalveolar root fractures: radiographic and histological study of 50 cases. *Journal of Oral Surgery*, **25**, 414–426

Jacobsen, I. and Zachrisson, B.U. (1975) Repair characteristics of root fractures in permanent anterior teeth. *Scandinavian Journal of Dental Research*, **83**, 355–364

Zachrisson, B.U. and Jacobsen, I. (1975) Long-term prognosis of 66 permanent anterior teeth with root fracture. *Scandinavian Journal of Dental Research*, **83**, 345–354

Chapter 9
Multiple injuries

M.E.J. Curzon and M.S. Duggal

On occasion, but fortunately rarely, dentists may have to deal with multiple injuries of the teeth and soft tissues. A combination of the following may be present:

- multiple tooth avulsions;
- pulp exposures together with luxations and/or avulsions (Figure 9.1);
- pulp exposures with severe tissue damage and swollen lips;
- alveolar fractures with or without luxations/avulsions.

These combinations of injuries can be very difficult to treat and in many cases may require admission to hospital for the necessary care to be carried out under a general anaesthetic. However, there are emergency measures that a dentist may, in practice, need to carry out in multiple injury cases.

As multiple injuries arise because of severe blows to the face, the authors' experience shows that the commonest causes are:

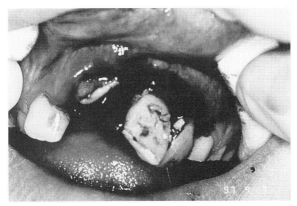

Figure 9.1 Photograph showing severe injuries to maxillary incisors resulting in complicated crown fractures and luxations

- **assaults** involving kicking or the use of blunt instruments to the face;
- **falls** onto the face from a height;
- **epileptic fits** or convulsions;
- **road traffic accidents** (RTAs).

In many of these instances there will almost certainly be legal implications and therefore, as noted many times before, detailed records using the trauma form are needed. Even in the event of epileptic fits or convulsions the authors have had to deal with cases where schools or carers have been sued for lack of proper care and attention which left an afflicted patient unsupervised when they fell over during a fit.

MULTIPLE TOOTH AVULSIONS

In these cases many teeth are knocked out. It is possible for all maxillary and mandibular incisors to be avulsed, although it is usually only one jaw that is affected. Thus 4–8 incisors can be presented to a dentist, hopefully these days in a cup of milk. These injuries can occur from a severe blow to the face such as a teenager being kicked in the face by a horse, violent assault with a brick, bat (baseball or cricket), golf club, etc., or during a convulsion (Figure 9.2). The authors have seen many such cases over the years.

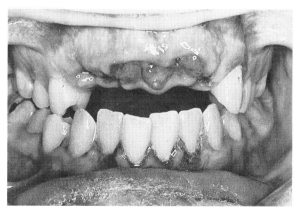

Figure 9.2 Photograph showing five maxillary anterior teeth avulsed during an epileptic fit in a teenager

The approach to be adopted is as follows:

- Take full **history** as quickly as possible.
- Make sure all **teeth are kept in milk**.
- Take **radiographs** of affected anterior teeth/sockets.
- **Check oral tissues** for damage, including the position of the alveolar cortical bone plates.
- **Debride** soft tissue lesions.
- Place **local analgesia**.
- **Reposition avulsed teeth** as soon as possible.
- **Splint** into position.
- Prescribe **antibiotics and analgesics** to be given immediately.
- Recommend **soft diet**.

However, in many of these cases the injuries are so extensive, particularly with displaced alveolar cortical plates, that it will be difficult in the extreme for a dentist in general dental practice to effectively reimplant, position and splint the teeth. Therefore in these cases the following approach should be adopted:

- Take brief **history**.
- Identify all avulsed teeth and **keep them in milk**.
- **Check oral tissues** for damage, including the position of the alveolar bone and the cortical plates.
- **Debride** soft tissue lesions.
- **Contact nearest consultant** in paediatric dentistry (or oral surgery) and advise them that the patient is being sent in for treatment.
- **Despatch patient** and accompanying person(s) to the nearest specialist by the fastest means possible.

The details given above have focused on avulsed teeth. However, there may be times when teeth have not been knocked out but have been luxated, sometimes at very odd angles. In these cases a dentist will find that the alveolar bone cortical plate has also been damaged and may well be very difficult to reposition. Treatment will require a general anaesthetic and hence a referral to a specialist.

PULP EXPOSURES TOGETHER WITH LUXATIONS AND/OR AVULSIONS

These cases are somewhat easier for the dental practitioner to handle, but they will require considerable chair time. These are instances where, rather than teeth being avulsed or luxated, the force of the blow has been dissipated by fracture of the crowns of several teeth.

Where one or two teeth have been involved, the approach is that described in Chapter 5. When a number of teeth are involved or where some teeth have pulp exposures and others are luxated, the approach requires a careful plan to ensure the best sequence of dental treatment.

The first priority, after taking a history and the appropriate radiographs, is to treat the pulp exposures. The rationale behind this is that the longer the exposed pulp tissue is open to infection, the poorer the prognosis. Hence the infected part of the pulp should be dealt with and the pulp tissue and dentine covered. The luxations can then be dealt with as described in Chapter 6. The step-by-step treatment of these cases is:

- Take full **history** as quickly as possible.
- Take **radiographs** of affected teeth.
- **Check oral tissues** for damage.
- **Debride** soft tissue lesions.
- Place **local analgesia**.
- Fit **rubber dam**.
- **Remove** exposed, infected pulp horns/coronal pulp tissue as necessary.
- Place **pulp capping** material.
- **Reposition** luxated tooth/teeth.
- **Splint** into position.
- Prescribe **antibiotics and analgesics** if required.
- Recommend **soft diet**.
- Arrange for **follow-up** appointments.

PULP EXPOSURES WITH SEVERE TISSUE DAMAGE AND SWOLLEN LIPS

Because there will have been extensive trauma resulting in the crown fractures and pulp exposures, there may well be considerable damage to the lips which very quickly become swollen. There may also be bruises, grazes and/or lacerations. Access to the fractured teeth becomes difficult because of the swollen lips.

The dentist is faced with the dilemma as to whether to deal with the injuries to the full extent necessary, treat the exposed pulps, leave them alone until the swellings have gone down or refer the patient for specialist care. However, as noted previously, exposed pulp tissue needs treating as quickly as possible, but the child may well be distressed and movement of the swollen lips will be painful.

If the damage is extensive and the patient is quite distressed, referral for specialist care may be in the child's best interest. The approach is as follows:

- **Palliative care** with coverage of the exposed pulp tissues so that they are protected until such time as a full treatment regimen can be implemented; this may require the use of **oral or inhalation (RA)** sedation if available and necessary.
- **Immediate referral** as quickly as possible.

If the former approach is selected, the treatment sequence is as follows:

- Take full **history** as quickly as possible.
- Take **radiographs** of affected teeth.
- **Check** all oral tissues for damage.
- **Debride** soft tissue lesions.
- **Cover** exposed, infected pulp horns/coronal pulp tissue with a protective agent, such as calcium hydroxide, with a layer of Vitrebond^R on top.
- Prescribe **antibiotics and analgesics** if required.
- Recommend **soft diet**.
- **Re-call** in 48 hours for proper treatment.

When the patient/child returns after 2 days, the swelling of the lips has usually gone down and so the teeth fractured with exposed pulps can be properly treated as described in the relevant chapters, according to the type of injury.

ALVEOLAR FRACTURES WITH OR WITHOUT LUXATIONS/AVULSIONS

Alveolar fractures, where the cortical plate of bone becomes separated and distorted away from the main cancellous bone, are difficult to treat. If the area of fracture is small, for example involving only one maxillary incisor, then it is easy to reposition the bone under local analgesia. Where several teeth are involved, the amount of manipulation needed to reposition the bone is such as to be very distressful for the patient, particularly children. This situation is even worse when the mandibular incisors are involved.

The approach in these cases depends on the extent of the injuries. Where only one or perhaps two maxillary incisors are involved, treatment can be carried out under local analgesia in the dental surgery. Where injuries are more extensive, a dentist should refer the patient as soon as possible to a specialist paediatric dentist or oral surgeon.

In cases of limited alveolar fracture and luxation/avulsion, the treatment approach is as follows:

- Take a full **history** as quickly as possible.
- Take **radiographs** of affected teeth.
- **Check** all oral tissues for damage.
- Give **local analgesia**.
- **Debride** soft tissue lesions.
- Carefully **reposition** the bony cortical plate that has been displaced.
- **Check the alveolus** is now sufficiently repositioned for an avulsed tooth to be reimplanted or a luxated tooth repositioned.
- **Replace** avulsed/luxated tooth/teeth.
- **Splint** into position.
- Prescribe **antibiotics and analgesics** if required.
- Recommend **soft diet**.

The patient should be re-called for the checking of the splint and commencement of the root canal therapy of the avulsed/luxated teeth as required.

SUMMARY

Multiple injuries involving several types of trauma to the teeth and soft tissues are difficult to treat in general dental practice. In most cases the best approach will be referral to a specialist paediatric dentist or oral surgeon. Where some form of immediate treatment is required, this should be as simple as possible, allowing for the swelling of the soft tissues, distress and discomfort of the patient.

Chapter 10

Soft tissue injuries

M.E.J. Curzom

It is very rare for injuries to the teeth not to also involve some soft tissue damage. In many cases such damage is minor and heals on its own. Also, such soft tissue damage does not usually interfere with the treatment of the damage to the tooth or teeth. However, when soft tissue injuries do occur they can be severe and require immediate attention. In rare cases the soft tissues require immediate treatment which necessitates leaving the repair of the teeth to a later date.

TYPES OF SOFT TISSUE INJURY

All the soft tissues may be involved and therefore should be systematically checked for the following:

- **Lips** – cuts in the lips, bruises, contusions, foreign particles, pieces of teeth, vermilion border injuries.
- **Frenum** – torn, cut as a result of a blow to the face.
- **Cheeks** – bites due to forcible closure of the jaws, tears, contusions.
- **Gingivae** – tears, crushing injuries.
- **Floor of the mouth** – penetrating wounds, lacerations, bruises.
- **Palate** – penetrating wounds, bruising.
- **Skin** – cuts, bruises, contusions.

The presence of foreign bodies should be particularly checked for. These will primarily be pieces of debris, such as dirt, as a result of the injury occurring outside in playing fields, playgrounds, etc. Injuries involving sports are often associated with dirt and debris becoming imbedded into the tissues. Another *foreign body* is a piece of a broken tooth from the same patient. This can be in the lips, but may also be found in other tissues. In the authors' experience, pieces of broken tooth have been found in a patient's knee. On other occasions we have noted pieces of tooth in the scalp arising from another child who was involved in a fight.

This indicates that when a tooth is noted as fractured, some effort should be made to find out where the broken pieces are. If not located then recheck the soft tissues. In Chapter 2, the technique of taking a radiograph of a lip is demonstrated and should be used whenever damage to the lips is noted. Besides pieces of tooth, this radiographic view will also show dirt and debris.

SOFT TISSUE DAMAGE AND TREATMENT

The following notes outline the approach to treatment of soft tissues.

Lips

Minor **crushing** damage from blows to the lip(s) against the teeth or bone usually requires only debridement and cleaning. Similarly, **bruising** of the lips without breaking of the mucous membrane or skin can be left to heal on its own.

Minor **cuts** of less than about 5 mm will normally heal on their own. If there is evidence of contamination the cut should be gently flushed with warm saline to remove particulate matter. Healing in children is rapid and the cut surface will soon close.

In older children, adolescents and young adults it may be necessary to suture the cut with fine resorbable 5–0 sutures. Larger cuts will definitely require suturing. In all cases local analgesia is indicated.

Frenum

A torn frenum is sometimes associated with trauma to the teeth and lips. In very young children it is often a sign of non-accidental injury (NAI) which is discussed later in Chapter 14. Sweeping blows to the face of a young child, as an adult lashes out with a hand, may rip the upper lip upwards so that tearing of the maxillary labial frenum occurs. This type of injury is not always associated with NAI, as such a blow can occur in fights. A detailed history will determine whether there is a possibility of NAI.

When a torn frenum occurs, the treatment is to suture the torn parts of the frenum together under local analgesia. In young children this may require a general anaesthetic.

Cheeks

Damage to the cheeks occurs when the teeth are slammed together during a fall on the ground or against another hard object, such as a table. Blows to the chin when the mouth is partially open may also cause this injury. The cheeks of young children are podgy and in the sudden closure of the teeth the cheek tissue becomes bitten, causing a linear laceration. In extreme cases the fat deposits of the cheek, or even muscle tissue, may extrude through the lesion.

Crushing damage to the cheek without any extrusion of cheek tissues may be left to heal after debridement. Any signs of foreign body contamination should be explored. Otherwise the tissue requires suturing using fine resorbable sutures.

Gingivae

Damage to the gingivae is a very common injury with trauma to the mouth and teeth. There may be only trauma to the gingivae and no other injuries, but more often the teeth have been damaged through displacement injuries which may tear the gingivae. There may well be multiple tears.

Before attempting to replace the gingivae, attention has to be given to replacing the displaced teeth, as described in previous chapters. Once the teeth have been repaired, repositioned and splinted, the gingivae should carefully be replaced, ensuring that the gingival cuff is carefully replaced to the damaged teeth. Minor tears will be retained in position and heal. Larger tears, particularly those going into the mucobuccal fold, will need suturing back into position. In order to ensure a good final result, the suturing should commence at the gingival margin.

Floor of the mouth

Children are sometimes involved in accidents when they have an object in their mouth. This might be a pencil, stick or pen, etc. The sudden blow drives the object deep into the mouth, penetrating the floor of the mouth or palate. The result is a tear.

The treatment is to suture the tear. However, this is often a complex injury which may involve the submandibular glands and lingual blood vessels. Repair of this type of injury may require that the child be placed under a general anaesthetic. Therefore, referral to a hospital is advised.

Very rarely, damage in the way of bruising to the floor of the mouth may be associated with NAI, where there has been sexual abuse with forcible oral sex. A detailed history is required and referral to a consultant in paediatric dentistry or paediatrician needed.

Palate

As noted above, penetrating injuries due to slim objects held in the mouth during a fall may cause wounds of the palate. Occasionally the object, pencil or pen, is lodged firmly in the palate and the child presents with it in place. These injuries also require the child be put to sleep with a general anaesthetic in order to repair the trauma effectively.

Skin

The skin to the face, particularly around the lips and on the cheeks, may be damaged during trauma. Minor cuts and lacerations may be repaired and held in place during primary healing with butterfly adhesive bandages.

Gaping holes will require suturing using microfilament sutures. As with a number of the soft tissue injuries discussed above, these will best be dealt with by referral to hospital.

SUMMARY

Soft tissue injuries are often associated with damage to the teeth. In the majority of cases these injuries will be minor and require only debridement and simple repair. More serious injuries, including gaping lacerations to the lips and cheek, and penetrating injuries to the floor of the mouth and palate, should be referred to a dental department of a hospital.

FURTHER READING

Davis, P.K.B. and Shaheen, O. (1995) Soft tissue injuries. In *Maxillo-Facial Injuries*, 2nd edn (edited by Rowe, N.L. and Williams, J.Ll). Churchill Livingstone, Edinburgh

Chapter 11
Splinting of traumatized teeth

S.A. Fayle

Traumatic injuries can result in loosening of teeth either by disruption of the periodontal ligament or by causing a root fracture. Appropriate splinting of traumatically loosened teeth allows them to be held in a stable position, which may assist healing, minimizes the risk of complications developing, avoids further disruption of the periodontal tissues, and improves patient comfort and confidence. Splints may also be used for a variety of other purposes, including maintaining stability after orthodontic treatment and for the stabilization of teeth compromised by periodontal disease, but this chapter will be confined to splinting following dento-alveolar trauma.

PRINCIPLES OF SPLINTING

The main aim of dental splinting after traumatic injuries is to support the damaged dental tissues, allowing optimal healing to occur. The type and duration of splinting therapy depends upon the exact nature of the dental injuries and the type of healing desired.

Damage to the periodontal ligament may heal by replacement resorption (ankylosis), a complication which is associated with a poor long-term prognosis (see Chapter 7). The risk of ankylosis increases with the severity of the periodontal insult, being particularly common following intrusive luxation and exarticulation, and less common in lateral and extrusive luxation. The risk of ankylosis developing is reduced by minimizing the period of splinting and using techniques which allow some degree of mobility of the injured teeth when in function.

Conversely, the healing of damaged dental hard tissues, following root fracture, for example, is thought to be facilitated by very rigid splinting of sufficient duration to allow an organized hard tissue repair to develop.

There are three different types of injury which require splinting:

- luxation;
- avulsion;
- horizontal root fracture.

The rationale for the splinting of these types of injury is given below.

Luxation

In luxation injuries the periodontal ligament is often severely disrupted. The main injury involves tearing of the periodontal ligament, usually accompanied by fracture of the associated alveolar bone. In addition, unless the injury is a simple extrusion (which is very rare) some areas of the periodontal ligament will have suffered a crushing injury. This will be most severe in **intrusive luxations**, where large areas of the periodontium may suffer irreversible damage secondary to crushing. These teeth are usually very firm at initial presentation and rarely require splinting, although orthodontic extrusion shortly after the injury may be indicated. As a consequence of the severe cellular damage, the periodontium of these teeth rarely undergoes normal healing.

Lateral and extrusive luxation injuries tend to result in less severe crush injuries, and normal healing of the periodontium can be anticipated in 60–90% of cases (Andreasen and Pedersen, 1985), depending upon the nature of the injury and the stage of apical development. There is a small but significant risk of replacement resorption (ankylosis), which requires that splinting should allow some physiological mobility and not be extended for longer than necessary (Oikarinen, 1988).

However, the damage to the crestal alveolar bone which frequently accompanies luxation can induce bony resorption of interdental and marginal bone during healing which may compromise the stability and safety of the injured tooth. Accordingly, initial splinting of luxated teeth should be maintained for 3 weeks, at which time the status of the surrounding alveolar bone should be reviewed radiographically and compared with the radiographic appearance at the time of the injury. If no bony resorption is present, the splint is then removed. If, however, resorption is visible radiographically 3 weeks after the time of the injury, splinting should be maintained for a further 3–4-week period (Andreasen and Andreasen, 1994).

Avulsion

Healing of the periodontium by replacement resorption and ankylosis is a frequent sequel to avulsion (sometimes also termed 'exarticulation injuries'). The risk of ankylosis becomes greater as the extra-alveolar time increases. Because of this, a splinting technique which maintains the tooth in the desired anatomical position but which also allows some degree of physiological mobility is preferred. Non-rigid splinting is thought to reduce the risk of ankylosis developing (Andersson *et al.*, 1985; Kristerson and Andreasen, 1983).

The optimum duration of splinting is 7–10 days. Longer periods should only be used if the tooth or teeth involved are still excessively loose at the end of this period.

Horizontal root fracture

It is generally agreed that the most desirable outcome following a horizontal root fracture injury is repair by hard tissue union between the coronal and apical fragments (see Chapter 8). For this to occur, the luxation of the coronal portion of the tooth, which frequently accompanies this type of injury, must be reduced so that the fractured surfaces are brought into close approximation, and then the tooth splinted in this position. The splint used needs to be rigid to prevent unwanted movement disturbing the healing tissues. Because of the length of time required for dentine and cementum-like tissues to form and organize, long periods of splinting are usually advocated, usually 12–14 weeks.

TYPES OF SPLINT

A large number of different splinting techniques have been used and described in the literature for the management of dento-alveolar trauma. Each of the more widely recognized techniques is described below, together with information about the indications for and the advantages and disadvantages of each approach. The main types used are now:

- composite/acrylic resin and arch wire;
- approximal composite/acrylic resin;
- composite/acrylic sausage;
- composite/acrylic nylon monofilament suture (fishing line);
- orthodontic brackets with sectional wire;
- sling suturing;
- vacuum-formed splints;
- removable acrylic resin plate;
- emergency splinting with limited equipment.

Composite/acrylic resin and arch wire

This type of splint is relatively easily constructed and allows the injured tooth or teeth to be splinted against adjacent teeth in the same arch. It is suitable for splinting single or multiple teeth, but may not be appropriate where adjacent teeth are unerupted, missing or injured.

Technique

The tooth/teeth to be splinted is/are repositioned (if necessary) and their crowns, together with the crowns of the teeth which are to support the splint, are cleaned, dried and isolated. Orthodontic wire of the desired gauge is selected and a piece is cut to length and shaped so that it will lie against the labial surfaces of the tooth/teeth to be splinted and at least one abutment tooth on either side (Figure 11.1).

The central area of each crown is then etched with phosphoric acid for 30 seconds, washed and dried. Bonding agent (unfilled resin or a proprietary enamel bonding system) is applied to a small circular area in the middle of the buccal surface of each crown (keeping well clear of the gingiva), followed by a blob of light cure composite resin. The wire is seated down into the composite resin which is then cured, starting with the outermost abutment teeth first. The composite resin on the tooth/teeth requiring splinting should be cured last. This allows for any final readjustment of the position of the damaged teeth prior to securing their final position. Further composite resin can be added to ensure that the wire is secure and a brush dipped in unfilled resin can be used to smooth the composite surface.

This type of splint can be used for both flexible and rigid splinting. For flexible splinting, a multi-strand orthodontic wire (e.g. twistflex) is most appropriate, although 0.5 mm diameter, or less, stainless steel wire may be used. Only one abutment tooth on either side is usually included, which also helps to maintain some degree of mobility.

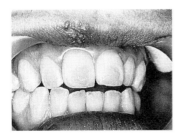

Figure 11.1 Photograph of first stage of placing a composite resin and wire splint. The teeth have been etched and blobs of composite placed

For rigid splinting, heavy-gauge round or square section orthodontic wire is used (0.8 mm diameter or greater) and at least two abutment teeth are included on either side wherever possible (Figure 11.2).

Modified acrylic resins designed for temporary crown/bridge construction may be used in place of composite resin. These will also bond to etched enamel, but with less strength enabling easier subsequent removal, but making them unsuitable for use with long-term rigid splinting. In addition, these materials are chemically cured, making them suitable for situations where specialized dental equipment is not available (see below in the section on 'Emergency out of hours splinting').

It is important to provide some protection for the airway during the construction and placement of wire splints. In many instances this can be achieved by using a prefabricated semi-rigid rubber dam, such as Dry Dam^R. Where this is not possible, the mouth can be protected with gauze, or floss can be tied around the splinting wire to allow its retrieval if dropped into the mouth.

Approximal composite/acrylic resin

This type of splint is quick and easy to place, as only one tooth requires splinting and directly adjacent uninjured teeth are available. The technique is simply to etch the approximal surfaces of the affected tooth and those of the adjacent teeth. A small amount of composite resin material is run into the embrasures and cured.

This is a very quick technique but has a disadvantage. Removal of the composite resin, once the splinting has been completed, is not easy and there is a risk of damaging the enamel surfaces of the teeth in stagnation areas.

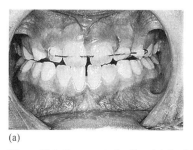
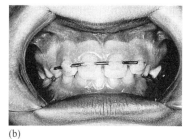

(a)   (b)

Figure 11.2 Placement of splint: (a) flexible splint; (b) rigid wire

Composite/acrylic sausage

This technique quickly produces a rigid splint using the minimum of materials and equipment (Figure 11.3). This makes it particularly suitable as a method of emergency or intermediate splinting, after hours or in hospital casualty departments, etc. The central areas of the buccal aspect of the crowns to be included in the splint are etched, as in the composite and wire splinting technique described above.

The teeth are supported in the desired position and a 'sausage' of composite resin, or acrylic crown and bridge material, is placed across the buccal surfaces of the affected teeth and, if necessary, cured.

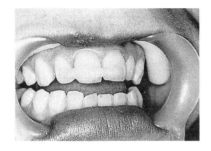

Figure 11.3 Photograph of composite resin sausage applied to stabilize maxillary anterior teeth

Composite/acrylic nylon monofilament suture (fishing line)

This clever idea enables flexible splints to be constructed without the need for wire-work. The teeth are prepared in the same way as above but, instead of a flexible wire, a short length of nylon monofilament suture or fishing line is used. A knot is tied in one end of the suture and the suture is wedged into an interproximal space distal to the last tooth to be included in the splint. After etching the teeth and placing blobs of composite/acrylic as before, the suture is pulled across the teeth and pushed into the composite/acrylic (Figure 11.4a). Once the composite/acrylic has been cured, the ends of the suture material are trimmed with suture removal scissors (Figure 11.4b).

Orthodontic brackets with sectional wire

Edgewise or straight-wire brackets and light wires may be used to produce flexible splinting. This technique is more involved than some of those previously described and will not result in a splint rigid enough for the treatment of root fractures, but it does allow for the reduction of displaced teeth by orthodontic forces, where desired.

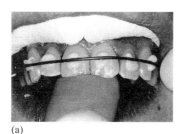
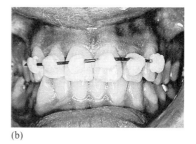

(a)   (b)

Figure 11.4 Emergency splint with composite and fishing line: (a) teeth etched and blobs of resin placed; fishing line secured by a knot in the distal interproximal space and laid across the composite resin for curing; (b) finished splint.

Sling suturing

Sling sutures are especially useful for the splinting of single teeth where no suitable abutment teeth for splint support is present (Figure 11.5).

Following administration of suitable local analgesia and repositioning of the tooth, heavy (2–0) nylon monofilament suture is passed through the interdental papilla on one side of the tooth, with as deep a bite as possible being taken when passing the needle through the tissues. The suture is then brought across the incisal edge of the tooth and the needle then passed deeply through the interdental papilla on the other side of the tooth and in the opposite direction as previously described. The suture is then once again looped over the incisal edge of the tooth, pulled tight and finally the two ends of the suture are knotted together (Figure 11.5).

In young teeth with pronounced mammelons, this arrangement is usually stable, but additional composite resin bulges can be constructed mesially and distally to prevent the suture from slipping off the incisal edge (Figure 11.5).

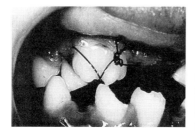

Figure 11.5 Photograph of maxillary anterior teeth stabilized with sling suturing. Sutures are placed to stabilize young incisors and composite resin used to prevent sutures slipping off

Vacuum-formed splints

Although they do have some limited value, and have been extensively used in the past, vacuum-formed splints have a number of disadvantages. Soft vacuum-formed splints do not offer sufficient support for luxated or avulsed (exarticulated) teeth, but can be used for some minor subluxations to help avoid further trauma or to give patients more confidence when eating, etc.

The vacuum-formed splint is extended over the alveolar mucosa and not cemented in place. As the splint is removable, oral hygiene should not be seriously compromised and the teeth are easily accessed for follow-up examination and special tests.

Rigid vacuum-formed splints can be used where multiple anterior teeth require splinting, and allow the rest of the arch to be used for stabilization. When used in this way the splints are constructed of acetate, trimmed to the level of the gingival margin and cemented in place with dental cement, usually zinc phosphate, as this is relatively easily removed when the splint is de-cemented.

The main **disadvantages** with vacuum-formed splints are that an accurate impression and laboratory facilities are required for construction. In addition, luxated or avulsed teeth need to be supported in the correct position during impression-taking if there is not to be a risk of the avulsed teeth being removed again with the set impression material. Although this can be achieved with a hook-shaped wire looped over the incisal edge, in practice this is quite difficult. It is also impossible to assess the occlusion accurately and the cemented type of splint can severely compromise gingival healing and health. Oral hygiene is also not easy to maintain and in many cases the vacuum-formed splint becomes foul.

In the authors' experience, **vacuum-formed splints frequently fail** to produce a satisfactory result and should be avoided, except in the specific situations detailed above.

Removable acrylic resin plate

This type of splint can provide flexible splinting and protection for one or more injured incisors. It has the advantage that it is removable, allowing access for oral hygiene and for follow-up examination/ special tests. However, it suffers from similar disadvantages to the vacuum-formed splints, in that an accurate impression of the teeth in the desired splinting position is required, laboratory facilities are needed and the occlusion is difficult to assess during splint construction and initial placement.

Emergency splinting with limited equipment

Hospital-based dentists, especially those on-call in accident and emergency departments, are frequently called upon to splint teeth in less than ideal conditions, where access to a comprehensively equipped dental surgery is not possible. There are a number of approaches which can be employed in such circumstances which enable effective splinting to be achieved. The metal foil and cement splint (Figure 11.6a) is still useful when other methods cannot be used. It is, however, only a very temporary measure (often only lasting for 24 hours or so). Injured teeth splinted in this way usually need more definitive splinting and often subsequently need repositioning. The foil splint should be placed using a thin mix of zinc oxide/eugenol cement, so as to make removal easier.

These emergency splints should only be used as a temporary measure until a better splinting technique is available. Thus the patient with a temporary or an emergency splint (see end of this chapter) must be seen again within 24 hours for a better and more appropriate splint to be fitted.

A similar, slightly more effective, splint can be made out of Stomahesive[R] bandage (Figure 11.6b). A suitably sized strip of bandage is cut from the square of material selected and adapted to the teeth and alveolus. This is easier if the bandage is dropped into warm water for a few seconds prior to placement. Although this may last for a few days, such splints are not reliable for definitive splinting, and can be messy to remove.

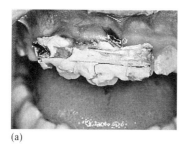

(a)

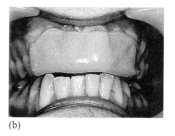

(b)

Figure 11.6 Examples of temporary splints: (a) metal foil splint; (b) Stomahesive bandage

EFFICIENT PLACEMENT OF SPLINT

Of the many types or methods of splints available, the best is that of a physiological splint that allows movement of the teeth during the healing process. At the same time, as noted in Chapter 1, it is imperative that the method used should be as simple as possible. Fitting of a splint in the dental chair can be staged so as to allow for other dental work to be carried out. In the technique described below, it is possible to place the local analgesia first and, while it is taking effect, another patient may be seen.

Once the local analgesia has taken effect, the next sequence of steps could be isolation, cleaning and etching the teeth. The splint is then quickly placed and, while the composite resin is curing, another patient can be attended to. Using this approach the normal running of the dental practice is not seriously disrupted by treating the trauma patient.

Technique for placement of physiological splints

- Following examination, radiographs and diagnosis, **local analgesia is administered** (if necessary).
- **Reposition** teeth to be splinted.
- Patient is asked to **bite onto a pad of gauze**, supporting the loosened tooth/teeth and isolating them from the mouth.
- A **dry dam**, **or rubber dam**, may be placed to isolate the affected teeth, or orthodontic **cheek retractors** used.
- If peri-oral injuries are serious this may not be possible, in which case cotton wool rolls may be used instead.
- **Twistflex wire** is taken and cut to the desired length.
- Clean **buccal surfaces** of the teeth to be included with a rubber cup and prophypaste.
- **Dry teeth** with dry, oil-free air from a three-way syringe.
- **Etch buccal surfaces** with phosphoric acid gel.
- After 30 seconds, **wash off the gel** using the three-way syringe and dry.
- Place **bobs of composite resin** in centre of facial surface of etched teeth.
- **Insert twistflex wire** into composite resin blobs and press into place.
- **Cure** composite resin, starting with outermost teeth and finishing with displaced or reimplanted tooth.

The above sequence of events is also shown in Figure 11.7.

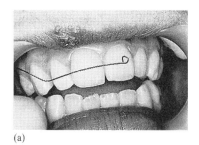

(a)

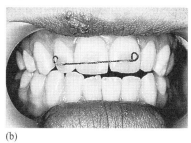

(b)

Figure 11.7 Placement of physiological splints: (a) twistflex wire cut and adapted to buccal surfaces of teeth to be splinted; (b) completed splint

EMERGENCY OUT OF HOURS SPLINTING

Equipment for placing emergency splints

With a little forward planning it is quite possible to be able to place effective rigid or flexible acrylic-based splints, and the technique for achieving this may be done with limited equipment (e.g. in the hospital casualty department or on a hospital ward). Based upon many years of experience of on-call after-duties, the authors have found the equipment listed below sufficient to cover the needs of emergency splinting.

Often the call that there is a child with damaged teeth comes in the early or late evening, between 6 and 10.00 p.m. It is the responsibility of every dentist to respond to such a call and to attend. Unfortunately very few A&E departments now have a dental surgery, so that emergency dental care has to be provided under less than ideal circumstances. In this case, dentists who are likely to be called for such eventualities should prepare by having an emergency dental kit available. This should be fitted out not only for trauma but also for toothaches (temporary dressing materials) and extractions (forceps, etc.).

The equipment required is as follows and can be carried in a fishing tackle plastic box very effectively (Figure 11.8):

- dressing kit of mirror, explorer, sharp excavator, flat plastic;
- temporary dressing material (IRM^R, Kalzinol^R, etc.);
- temporary crown and bridge cement (e.g. Protemp IIr);
- cheek retractors;
- rubber gloves;
- phosphoric acid etching gel;
- brush to place etchant;
- 50 ml syringe filled with sterile water with an intravenous cannula attached;
- cotton wool rolls;
- gauze;
- local analgesia equipment, topical benzocaine, 30 g needles, self-aspirating syringe;
- extraction forceps as used (76S is recommended);
- wooden tongue blades;
- oxygen mask tubing for attachment to oxygen cylinder/supply.

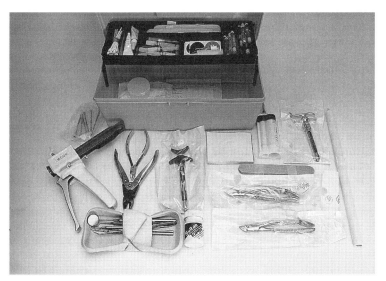

Figure 11.8 Emergency box and dental equipment for after-hours treatment of dental trauma and other dental emergencies

Method

- Following examination and diagnosis, **local analgesia is administered** (if necessary).
- **Reposition** teeth to be splinted.
- Patient is asked to **bite onto a pad of gauze**, supporting the loosened tooth/teeth and isolating them from the mouth.
- Insert cheek retractor to **hold the lips away** from the teeth.
- If perioral injuries are serious this will not be possible, in which case **cotton wool rolls** may be used instead.
- **Clean buccal surfaces** of the teeth to be included with a cotton wool roll.
- Sometimes it helps to **clean the teeth** with a cotton swab dampened with spirits (isopropyl alcohol, etc.).
- **Dry teeth** with a stream of oxygen from the oxygen mask tubing.
- **Etch buccal surfaces** with phosphoric acid gel.
- After 30 seconds, **wash off the gel** using the 50 ml syringe which has the flexible end of an intravenous cannula attached (inner needle discarded).
- Use **suction**, but if suction is not available the patient should be seated upright with a kidney dish below their chin.
- **Change the gauze** and dry the teeth again with a stream of oxygen.
- **Check** to ensure the tooth is repositioned correctly and if necessary it is supported by a finger.
- **Place temporary crown material** (Protemp), applied as a thin sausage across the buccal surfaces and patted into place with a plastic instrument.
- The material is most easily applied directly from a **self-mixing delivery system** (e.g. Garant gun). (Note: If this type of delivery system is used, the first material which is extruded is often incompletely mixed and should be discarded.)

The sequence of events is shown in Figure 11.9.

After placing the temporary splint, and before final setting of the material, a gloved finger should be used to flatten the material and ensure a smooth finish. The patient should then be given after-care instruction which should include directions for seeking more permanent long-term care as soon as possible.

While these temporary splints can last successfully for the required 7–10 days, they often de-bond after 48 hours. A better physiological splint, as described above, should be placed as soon as possible. It is advisable that the patient (child) should be advised to attend their own dentist at the next available opportunity, preferably the next day, for

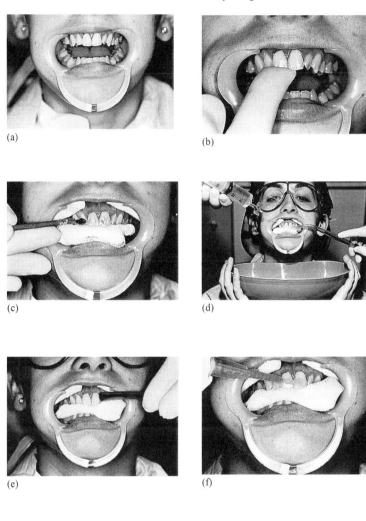

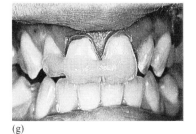

Figure 11.9 Emergency splinting:
(a) local analgesia is given and cheek
retractors placed; (b) displaced teeth
repositioned; (c) teeth cleaned, isolated
and etching gel applied; (d) teeth washed;
(e) teeth dried with stream of oxygen and
checked for position; (f) sausage of
temporary crown and bridge material
applied across teeth to be splinted;
(g) final temporary splint in position

the splint either to be checked or replaced with a more stable one, as described earlier in this chapter.

SUMMARY

Modern adhesive materials have ensured that rapid splinting of displaced teeth can be effectively carried out quickly to enhance the successful outcome of reimplanted or repositioned teeth. It is suggested that an effective emergency splint can quickly be fabricated with a minimal amount of portable dental equipment and materials.

REFERENCES

Andreasen, J.O., Lindskoe, S., Blomlof, L., Hedstrom, K.-G. and Hammarstrom, L. (1985) Effect of masticatory stimulation on dentoalveolar ankylosis after experimental tooth replantation. *Endodontics and Dental Traumatology*, **1**, 13–16

Andreasen, J.O. and Pedersen, V. (1985) Prognosis of luxated permanent teeth: the development of pulp necrosis. *Endodontics and Dental Traumatology*, **1**, 207–220

Andreasen, J.O. and Andreasen, F.M. (1994) *Textbook and Colour Atlas of Traumatic Injuries to the Teeth*, 3rd edn. Munksgaard, Copenhagen

Kristerson, L. and Andreasen, J.O. (1983) The effect of splinting upon periodontal and pulpal healing after autotransplantation of mature and immature permanent incisors in monkeys. *International Journal of Oral Surgery*, **12**, 239–249

Oikarinen, K. (1988) Comparison of the flexibility of various methods of tooth fixation. *Journal of Oral and Maxillofacial Surgery*, **17**, 125–127

Chapter 12
Restoration of fractured teeth

K.J. Toumba

Frequently, apart from minor infractions, most fractured incisors will require an immediate, preferably semi-permanent, restoration. This is an area of dental treatment for trauma which is most often neglected or poorly carried out. The result is that many fractured teeth die unnecessarily when the simplest type of effective restoration would have protected the dentine. The objective of this chapter is to emphasize the need for the semi-permanent restoration of teeth and to give some advice on methods.

In the authors' experience, the treatment of fractured teeth with dentine or dentine/pulp exposures is to place a blob of glass ionomer cement on the fractured tooth and send the patient away. In nearly all cases this type of temporary restoration comes off, usually within a few days. The re-exposed dentine (and pulp) becomes contaminated and leads to death of the pulp tissues. Research by Ravn (1981a–c) showed that in teeth with extensive mesial or distal fractures, not adequately protected, some 54% developed pulpal necrosis. In contrast, of a group of similarly fractured teeth with good dentine coverage, only 8% developed pulpal necrosis.

Therefore, it is essential in treating any fractured tooth with dentine exposure to ensure that a good semi-permanent restoration is immediately placed. Such a restoration must be extensive enough to seal all exposed dentine completely. The restoration must also be sufficient to last for some years until a permanent restoration is appropriate.

TYPES OF TEMPORARY RESTORATION

Fractured teeth will require an immediate restoration with one of the following:

- enamel fracture – restored with composite resin build-up;
- enamel–dentine fracture – covered with Dycal[R], Vitrebond[R], Dyract[R] or composite resin;

- large enamel–dentine fracture – protection for the dentine plus composite resin;
- pulpal exposure – protection for pulp capping plus semi-permanent composite resin crown;
- large crown fracture – complete coverage composite resin crown.

It cannot be emphasized too strongly that some form of restoration must be placed. Even the smallest exposure of dentine in a young permanent tooth opens up dentinal tubules to infection and may lead to pulp death. It is very tempting for a busy dentist to dismiss small dentinal exposures as trivial and not requiring any protection.

The authors have seen many children over the years, who attend with minor fractures of the maxillary incisors, presenting with stained and decayed dentine of an old fracture. Sensibility (vitality) tests often indicate that the tooth is dead and in too many cases the presenting symptom is an abscess.

The answer is always to cover the exposed dentine as quickly as possible using a restoration that will seal and protect the dentine and, therefore, the pulp from further contamination.

TECHNIQUE FOR EXPOSED DENTINE

- **Isolate** tooth with cotton wool rolls, Dry Dam[R] or rubber dam.
- Gently **clean** exposed dentine with rubber cup and a thin slurry of prophylaxis paste.
- **Dry** tooth.
- **Cover** exposed dentine with proprietary calcium hydroxide or Vitrebond[R].
- **Build up** fractured enamel with composite resin to restore contour.
- **Reshape** incisors, if necessary, to improve aesthetics.

The coverage of the dentine by a protective material is important. As noted above, just to cover with a drop of Dycal[R] is not enough as it will always come off, usually within days. The young dentine with open tubules will inevitably become infected. Coverage with a composite resin material is therefore essential. If carefully placed and finished, such semi-permanent restorations may become permanent and last for years. An example is shown in Figure 12.1a, where teeth 11 and 21 were fractured in an 8-year-old boy and restored within 3 hours as a semi-permanent measure using celluloid crown forms. At follow-up 1 month later (Figure 12.1b), the restorations were sound. Not seen again for some 13 years, the restorations were found to be

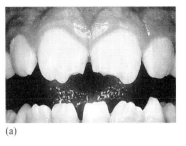
(a)

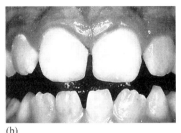
(b)

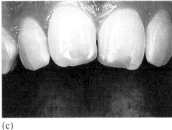
(c)

Figure 12.1 Repair of enamel–dentine fracture: (a) photograph showing fractured teeth 11 and 21; (b) initial dentine protection and composite resin repair; (c) the teeth 13 years after repair

still in place, albeit slightly discoloured, and showing signs of wear (Figure 12.1c). The patient declined to have them replaced.

SMALL ENAMEL–DENTINE FRACTURES

To ensure that the composite resin stays in place and maintains the contour of the tooth, the enamel edges should be trimmed to a straight line and the enamel bevelled. This will enhance the retention of the resin. Even small enamel–dentine fractures should be restored (Ravn, 1981c).

A useful tip is to use an Odus-Pella[R] celluloid crown form. While this involves some additional cost, for the crown form, it is worth while because of the superior restoration that is obtained. The crown form is selected for the appropriate size. However, old unusable sizes can also be selected which uses up old stock. The crown form is cut across diagonally to produce a form that will more than cover the fractured surface (Figure 12.2). A small hole is punched in the corner of the incisal edge.

After cleaning, the exposed dentine is protected, as described above. The enamel is etched, washed and dried. The cut crown form is then filled with composite resin fitted to the fractured tooth and cured. Once set, the composite resin is trimmed and smoothed with Baker–Curson burs and Soflex discs in the normal way.

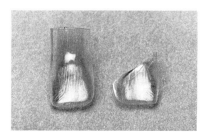

Figure 12.2 Crown form before and after trimming

LARGE ENAMEL–DENTINE FRACTURES

These are restored in the same way as for minor fractures, as discussed above. However, attempts to restore these fractured teeth with small composite repairs often fail. Full crown coverage is therefore essential.

Rationale for full crown coverage

The main reason for failure, if a small restoration is placed, is that a dentist tries to restore only the lost piece of crown. Teeth that have been fractured once are always subject to further fracture. This may be because the teeth are proclined (Class II division I malocclusion, before orthodontic treatment) or the child is *accident-prone*.

Another reason is that with large fractures the amount of enamel available for bonding is small in relation to the amount of tooth lost. It is therefore very easy for the small piece of composite resin, inadequately bonded to enamel, to be knocked off.

When a temporary restoration becomes knocked off, the dentine will be exposed yet again to bacterial contamination. In young permanent teeth the dentinal tubules are very wide and the dentine protective material does not adhere very well. When a temporary restoration is lost, the protection is soon also lost. Ingress of bacteria down the dentinal tubes happens very quickly, leading to pulpal necrosis, pulp death and abscess formation. Complete and prolonged sealing of the exposed dentine is therefore essential. The protective restoration must last securely for many months or years or until the dentist is certain of radiographic and clinical success.

The solution to this problem is a full-coverage composite resin crown using the celluloid crown form. The procedure for this is as follows:

- **Isolate** tooth with cotton wool rolls, Dry Dam^R or rubber dam.
- Gently **clean** exposed dentine and enamel with rubber cup and a thin slurry of prophylaxis paste.
- **Dry** tooth.
- **Cover** exposed dentine with proprietary calcium hydroxide and/or Vitrebond^R.
- **Select celluloid crown** for fractured tooth.
- Cut and **trim crown form** to fit over the *whole* crown.
- **Puncture small holes** in incisal edge of crown form.
- **Etch** enamel.
- **Wash** and thoroughly **dry**.
- **Fill** crown form with composite resin and fit over fractured tooth.
- **Trim** off excess resin.
- **Cure** composite resin, both palatally and buccally.
- **Strip off** celluloid crown form.
- Give a final trim and **polish** to the cured crown with Baker–Curson burs and Soflex discs.
- **Reshape** incisors, if necessary, to improve aesthetics.

Dentists should not be tempted to 'save time' by not providing full coverage. The time saved is lost at a later date by the extensive amount of chairside time required for the endodontics with an infected root canal. It may be that temporary small composite resin or glass ionomer cement can be placed on the day of the fracture, but the full crown coverage must be provided within 24 hours.

PULPAL EXPOSURE

The comments made above concerning sealing of the damaged tooth from outside contamination equally apply to complicated fractures involving the pulp. As soon as possible the fractured crown should be encased in a full-coverage composite resin crown. Once fabricated, an access cavity is cut palatally in order to commence the endodontics that are required (see Chapter 5). It is imperative that the root canal is sealed from bacterial ingress.

FRACTURED CROWN

Where nearly all of the crown of an incisor has been fractured off, and is available, it is possible to re-bond the crown if it is in one piece. Where the crown has been lost, an alternative approach is required.

It is feasible to reattach a fractured crown fragment, or even a whole crown, with the excellent dentine bonding systems that are now available (Scotch Bond[R], etc.). However, few long-term studies on the success of this technique have been reported. There is also a tendency for the reattached fragment to become opaque or discoloured and to require further restorative intervention. While the authors have on occasion used the technique of crown reattachment, described below, its success is not good. With so many excellent composite resin materials available, it is probably better not to waste too much time attempting to reattach a crown, but rather to proceed to use a celluloid crown form and build up a proper semi-permanent restoration.

Re-bonding a fractured crown

If a dentist decides that re-bonding a fractured crown is the best approach at the time, the technique is as follows:

- **Check the fit** of the crown fragment.
- Check the **vitality** of the tooth.
- **Clean fragment** and tooth with pumice–water slurry.
- Isolate tooth/teeth with **rubber dam**.
- **Fix the crown fragment** to a gutta-percha or sticky wax stick to facilitate handling and positioning of the crown fragment.
- **Etch** enamel on both fracture surfaces for 30 seconds and extend etch to 2 mm from fracture line on both tooth and fragment.
- **Wash** tooth and fragment for 15 seconds.
- **Dry** both tooth and fragment for 15 seconds.
- **Apply dentine primer** to both surfaces and dry for 20–30 seconds.
- **Apply dentine bonding agent** to both surfaces, then lightly blow away any excess; light cure for 10 seconds.
- **Place** appropriate shade of composite resin over both surfaces.
- **Position fragment**, remove excess composite resin.
- **Cure** palatally and labially for 60 seconds.
- **Trim** and remove any further excess composite resin with sandpaper discs.
- Remove a 1 mm **gutter of enamel** on each side of the fracture line, both labially and palatally, to a depth of 0.5 mm using a small round or pear-shaped diamond bur; the finishing line should be irregular in outline.
- **Etch** the newly prepared enamel, wash, dry, apply fresh composite resin, **cure and finish**.

FINAL RESTORATION OF FRACTURED TEETH

The final restoration of a fractured tooth can only be carried out once the dentist is confident that the immediate and medium-term treatment has been successful. In some cases this may be several years. A carefully prepared and cured composite resin crown, using the celluloid crown form, will last for a long time and its aesthetics may well be acceptable under the circumstances.

A dentist should not be rushed into a final restoration by a parent or guardian simply because of the aesthetics. Indeed, it is sometimes advisable not to produce a crown of perfect aesthetics purely to ensure that the patient returns for follow-up appointments. Radiographic and clinical success needs to have been achieved before a final restoration is placed.

Depending on the size of the lost crown tissue, it is usually advisable to make use of composite resin restorations as much as possible. The modern composite resins are of excellent durability and aesthetics. In the authors' experience, most crown fractures can best be restored with a simple technique to provide a long-lasting restoration. However, larger crown fractures may require other forms of retention such as laboratory-formed porcelain or porcelain bonded to metal post crowns. These latter restorations are expensive and are best used only once a successful outcome of the treatment of the fractured tooth has been assured.

SUMMARY

It is essential to ensure that any fracture exposing dentine, or dentine and pulp, is immediately and properly restored. Semi-permanent restorations using celluloid crown forms and composite resins are the treatment of choice. The most important aspect of restoration of fractured teeth is sealing of the dentine and pulp tissue from outside contamination. This can only be achieved by the use of semi-permanent, well-made restorations.

REFERENCES AND FURTHER READING

Andreasen, J.O. and Andreasen, F.M. (1990) *Essentials of Traumatic Injuries to the Teeth*. Munksgaard, Copenhagen

Munksgaard, E.C., Hojtved, L., Jorgensen, E.H., Andreasen, J.O. and Andreasen, F.M. (1991) Enamel–dentin crown fractures bonded with various bonding agents. *Endodontics and Dental Traumatology*, **7**, 73–77

Ravn, J.J. (1981a) Follow-up study of permanent incisors with enamel cracks as a result of acute trauma. *Scandinavian Journal of Dental Research*, **89**, 117–123

Ravn, J.J. (1981b) Follow-up study of permanent incisors with enamel fractures as a result of acute trauma. *Scandinavian Journal of Dental Research*, **89**, 213–217

Ravn, J.J. (1981c) Follow-up study of permanent incisors with enamel–dentin fractures as a result of acute trauma. *Scandinavian Journal of Dental Research*, **89**, 355–365

Chapter 13

Injuries to the primary dentition: diagnosis and treatment modalities

E.A. O'Sullivan

Injuries to primary dentition are common and it has been estimated that up to 30% of pre-school children can be affected (Andreasen and Ravn, 1972). Trauma to the primary teeth occurs frequently, probably because young infants are unstable on their feet as they start to walk and then, in running around with their new found mobility, accidents happen which result in damaged primary teeth.

The roots of the primary teeth are in close relationship to developing permanent successors and therefore the force of any blow to the primary teeth can easily be transmitted to the underlying developing permanent dentition. In addition, infection arising subsequent to a primary tooth injury may damage the successional tooth. The treatment strategy after injury in the primary dentition is, therefore, dictated by a concern for the safety of the permanent dentition.

Prevalence

- Varies from 11% to 30% (often not reported).
- Most common between 1.5–2.5 years.
- Owing to the resilient bone surrounding the primary teeth, injuries are usually confined to supporting structures – avulsions, luxations, etc.

Aetiology

- Falls, collisions or bumps as a child starts walking.
- Physical abuse (non-accidental injury, see Chapter 14).

Assessment

- As for permanent teeth, but often there are difficulties due to lack of cooperation of the child.
- Sensibility (vitality) tests are unreliable.
- Radiographic examination – the easiest method is to take an

anterior oblique occlusal view using a periapical film, or an anterior occlusal film.

Sometimes a child-sized bitewing (Figure 13.1) film can be usefully used in a small mouth, or lateral oblique films can be used where a child finds it difficult to accept radiographic films placed in the mouth.

SOFT TISSUE INJURIES

These are common in the case of trauma to the primary dentition, owing to displacement of a tooth or teeth (Figure 13.2). In nearly all cases, the level of treatment required is minimal.

The treatment required is as follows:

- **Wash** the area of soft tissue injury with water or normal saline.
- **Suture**, if necessary, with local analgesia.
- Consider **antibiotic** coverage for 5–7 days.
- Check **anti-tetanus** status.
- **Recall** for a review after 7–10 days.

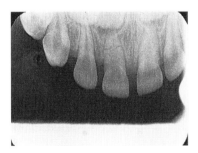

Figure 13.1 Radiograph showing use of a child-sized bitewing taken to assess damage to the maxillary primary incisors.

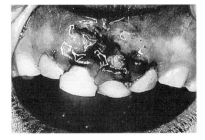

Figure 13.2 Photograph of trauma with soft tissue injuries to primary dentition

TREATMENT APPROACHES

Tooth fractures

A preliminary question is: should the injured primary tooth be saved? To answer this, the factors to consider are:

- Possible damage to **permanent tooth** or teeth.
- Patient **cooperation**.
- **Parental attitude**.
- Amount of **root remaining**.

There are a number of different types of injury to primary teeth, which can be classified as follows:

- **Fractures** to the crown or root of the primary tooth.
- **Luxation** or displacement injury.
- **Damage** to the permanent successor.

Treatment aims for primary teeth

- To prevent injury to the permanent successor.
- To save the primary tooth or teeth if compatible with the above aim.
- To restore tooth and aesthetics, if this is possible, with the least amount of active treatment compatible with the child's cooperation.

Diagnosis

The diagnosis of fractures or displacement injuries to the primary teeth is exactly the same as that for the permanent teeth. Thus, a full examination, as far as the child's cooperation will allow, should be carried out and the details recorded on the trauma form. Fractures of the enamel and dentine should be noted and also whether any fracture involves the pulp of the tooth or teeth. Fractures very close to the nerve should be considered as pulp exposures.

Radiographs

As for permanent teeth, suitable radiographs should be taken such as those described above and shown in Figure 13.1. Children with tooth fractures are often very young and may well not be cooperative enough to allow radiographs to be taken. The dentist must use his or her judgement to decide what is in the best interests of the child. Where possible it is always desirable to obtain a radiograph showing the crown and roots of the affected tooth or teeth. It may be necessary to carry this out at a review visit when the child is less upset.

Treatment approaches

The cooperation of the child is again a major factor here. If the child is distressed, very young and possibly in acute pain, little treatment may be possible. When a child is very uncooperative and in pain or the traumatized teeth are interfering with the occlusion, a general anaesthetic may be necessary. Alternatively, oral sedation can be useful and effective in very young children.

The treatment that should be carried out, if the child is cooperative, is as follows:

Enamel fractures

- Small chip – leave or smooth off rough edge.
- Larger chip – restore with composite resin.
- Review – as often there has also been a luxation injury.

Enamel–dentine fractures

- Protect pulp with calcium hydroxide or glass ionomer lining material.
- Restore with composite resin, or use a strip crown technique as described by Pollard and Fayle (1995).

Whole crown fractures

Whole crown fractures with large exposures of pulp are rare and in most cases extraction will be indicated. However, in some cases there will be a need to restore such a fractured incisor. This might be because of aesthetics. Where restoration is important, for whatever reason, the approach will be to treat the exposed pulpal tissue and to restore the crown. The prognosis for the pulp treatment will be assessed on the time elapsed since the fracture occurred. As with permanent teeth, the longer the time of pulp exposure the less likely for vital tissue to remain.

In these cases the dentist can carry out a pulpotomy or pulpectomy. In either case the medicament of choice will be formocresol followed by pure zinc oxide and eugenol, as described by Duggal and Curzon (1995).

Treatment of whole crown fractures

Whole crown fractures may be slight or extensive. Depending on how much tooth tissue is affected, the treatment options are:

- coronal pulpotomy and strip crown;
- pulpectomy and strip crown;
- extraction.

The techniques required here have been well described elsewhere (Duggal and Curzon, 1995; Pollard and Fayle, 1995).

Root fractures

Root fractures account for about 3% of traumas to the primary teeth. A periapical radiograph is required, as described earlier (Figure 13.1). Under no circumstances should an attempt be made to remove any apical root fragments as the risk of damage to the underlying permanent tooth crowns is high with instrumentation. The coronal fragment can be removed with forceps.

The success of the treatment approach will be:

- dependent on how stable the coronal fragment is; and
- the more coronal the fracture the worse the prognosis;
- it is often best to extract the coronal portion, but leave the apical portion to resorb.

DISPLACEMENT INJURIES TO PRIMARY TEETH

Avulsions

Never attempt to reimplant primary teeth

Because of the danger of damaging the underlying permanent teeth, no attempt should be made to reimplant an avulsed primary incisor. It is impossible to relocate the tooth accurately and there is great danger in pushing the primary incisor too far into the soft alveolar bone. A space maintainer/partial denture may be used to improve aesthetics if there is strong parental demand. In these rare cases, small fixed appliances may be fitted as a type of 'bridge' to replace the lost tooth. The reader is referred to textbooks of paediatric dentistry for the techniques required under these circumstances (McDonald and Avery, 1994).

Luxation injuries

Luxation injuries are common in small children, and primary teeth can be very easily displaced to the most bizarre angles. However, in most cases the displacement is slight and repositioning may be attempted. Where there is gross displacement, the injury should be treated as for an avulsion and the tooth extracted.

Many injuries to the primary incisors of small children involve some degree of displacement. Toddlers fall and hit their teeth on furniture or other objects and in the process the teeth are moved or displaced from their sockets.

The treatment is as follows:

- If slight and a tooth is not at risk of coming out of the socket spontaneously, **leave**, **advise a soft diet** and give oral hygiene instruction.
- If palatally displaced it may be possible to **gently reposition manually**, and monitor for loss of vitality and mobility.
- If the tooth does not show an improvement in mobility over the next 2 weeks, so that it becomes markedly looser in its socket, it should be **extracted**.
- If a radiographic examination reveals that the luxated primary incisor has been pushed into the developing permanent tooth, the primary tooth should be **extracted**.

Intrusion injuries

Intrusion injuries are also very common in infants when they fall and hit their front maxillary teeth on furniture as they learn to walk. In some instances a maxillary incisor or incisors may be completely intruded. The approach to treatment for these teeth is largely to establish where they are in the alveolus and then to leave them alone.

The treatment approaches are:

- Intruded teeth should be allowed to **re-erupt spontaneously**.
- If radiographic examination reveals **any pathology**, the tooth (teeth) should be **extracted**.
- If more than three-quarters of the crown has intruded, the tooth should be monitored.
- A **lateral radiograph**, such as that used for soft tissues (see Figure 2.5), should be taken to determine the position of the primary tooth in relation to the permanent successor.
- If the primary tooth is very close or touching the permanent tooth, the primary tooth should be **extracted**.

Extrusion injuries

Extrusion injuries which occur in the primary dentition usually interfere with the occlusion. Therefore, extraction is usually indicated.

- If extrusion is less than 1–2 mm, leave and monitor.
- If extrusion is more than 2 mm, the tooth will almost certainly have lost its vitality and therefore should be extracted.

MONITORING INJURIES TO PRIMARY TEETH

It is imperative to monitor and follow up all injuries to the primary dentition, no matter how apparently minor:

- All injuries to primary teeth should be monitored at 1 week, 1 month, 3 months, 6 months and 1 year, then at yearly intervals, until exfoliation.
- If periapical pathology occurs, the tooth should be extracted.
- Discoloration of primary teeth is not always an indicator of loss of vitality.
- Sensiblity testing in very young children is difficult, so that discoloured primary teeth should be monitored carefully for pathological changes.

Discoloration of a traumatized primary incisor is not an indication for extraction. Such incisors can remain in situ until exfoliation without any problems. Many such teeth regain a normal colour. The advice to parents is to leave the tooth (teeth) as it is. However, the parent should check weekly for the presence of a chronic abscess (gum boil) by retracting the upper lip and checking the condition of the free gingivae. This examination technique should be demonstrated to the parent.

Injury to permanent successors

Traumatic injuries to developing teeth can influence their future growth and maturation, usually leaving a child with a permanent deformity. The injuries to the developing teeth can be classified as follows:

- White or brown **discoloration** of the permanent tooth with or without hypoplastic enamel defects.
- **Dilaceration of the crown** of the tooth – causes eruption disturbance or failure.

- **Dilaceration of the root** of the tooth – causes eruption disturbance or failure.
- **Odontome**-like formation.
- **Root duplication**.
- Partial or total **failure of root development**.
- **Total failure** of tooth development.

The diagnosis of dilacerations of the permanent teeth (usually incisors) is difficult. In the presence of the primary dentition of a young child, any deformity of the growing permanent tooth will most likely not be seen. At a later stage of development, when the root of the permanent incisor is growing, the dilaceration may be diagnosed from a periapical radiograph (Figure 13.3). Often the first indication of a problem is the failure of the permanent tooth to erupt. Where a permanent incisor is markedly dilacerated, the tooth will ultimately need extracting. Sometimes the damage from the intruded primary incisor may be sufficient to cause a lack of development of the permanent tooth (Figure 13.3).

The prevalence of such disturbances, secondary to dental injuries in the primary dentition, ranges from 12% to 69%, according to different studies.

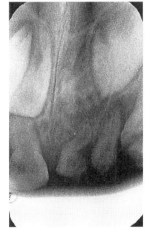

Figure 13.3 Radiograph showing dilaceration of a primary incisor (61) due to trauma very soon after eruption of this tooth and before root development was completed. The damage to the underlying permanent incisor (21) has led to failed development of the crown and root leaving a 'ghost' tooth

SUMMARY

Trauma to the primary dentition is very common and frequently involves primary maxillary incisors. Treatment of enamel and enamel–dentine fractures is palliative. Pulp exposures usually require extraction unless there are very good reasons to retain the tooth. Avulsed primary incisors should *not* be reimplanted. Intruded teeth should be left to re-erupt. Regular monitoring is needed to diagnose possible damage to the developing permanent incisors.

REFERENCES

Andreasen, J.O. and Ravn, J.J. (1972) Epidemiology of traumatic dental injuries to primary and permanent teeth in a Danish population sample. *International Journal of Oral Surgery*, **1**, 235–239

Duggal, M.S. and Curzon, M.E.J. (1995) Pulp therapy for primary teeth. In *Restorative Techniques in Paediatric Dentistry*. Martin Dunitz, London

McDonald, R.E. and Avery, D.R. (1994) Managing space problems. In *Dentistry for the Child and Adolescent*, 6th edn. C.V. Mosby, St Louis

Pollard, M.A. and Fayle, M.A. (1995) Strip crowns for primary incisors. In *Restorative Techniques in Paediatric Dentistry*. Martin Dunitz, London

Chapter 14

Non-accidental injuries: diagnosis and dento-legal aspects of care

E.A. O'Sullivan and J.F. Tahmassebi

Definition

Various words have been used over the years to describe physical trauma to a child. The most commonly used term is now non-accidental injury (NAI), but the condition is also known as *child abuse* or *baby battering*. NAI is defined as when a child is treated by an adult in a way that is unacceptable to their culture at a given time. It involves the physical trauma to a child by beating with the hands, and the use of instruments such as sticks, tools, knives, whips, etc. Injuries include burns and scalds and any other types of physical trauma. It has been reported that in over 50% of cases of NAI there are associated dental injuries (Becker *et al.*, 1978); therefore it is important that dentists are aware of its occurrence and have a knowledge of the presenting symptoms.

Physical NAI is the commonest form of child abuse and all professionals who deal with children in any capacity must be aware of its existence. All dentists should be able to diagnose possible cases of NAI, presenting as trauma to the teeth or oral cavity, and should know how to report cases to the appropriate agencies for further investigation.

In dentistry there is also the consideration that neglect of the teeth, in a very young child, such that they are grossly decayed but not cared for, constitutes a form of abuse (Hobbs and Winn, 1996). It is now thought by many paediatric dentists that such cases should be reported to the social services, just as a dentist should report a child who has attended their surgery with trauma to the teeth of suspicious origin (Becker *et al.*, 1978). In defining neglect we would describe it as occurring in pre-school children presenting an extensively decayed dentition involving more than two-thirds of the primary teeth and where there is no evidence or history that the parent or carer has attempted to attend a dentist with the child for care of the broken-down teeth. Obviously this is likely to be a controversial subject, as the borderline between dental decay of a number of teeth and neglect is ill-defined.

Nevertheless in the authors' experience, cases of dental neglect are usually quite clear. Children suffering from dental neglect present with severely broken-down black/brown stumps of teeth and no effort has been made to seek care for the child.

Prevalence

The 1986 survey by the National Society for the Prevention of Cruelty to Children (NSPCC), in the UK, reported that in that year in England and Wales 9500 children were physically injured, 6330 were sexually abused and approximately four children died every week as a result of NAI. About half the children are under the age of 5 years. Children under 2 years of age are most at risk of physical abuse, and in most age groups boys are more commonly abused than girls. Teenage girls are abused more frequently than boys of the same age. Approximately 33% of physically abused children suffer re-injury.

Aetiology

NAI is more common in the following situations:

- lower socio-economic groups;
- young parents;
- parents of lower intelligence;
- marital instability;
- history of NAI of the parents themselves when children;
- poor tolerance and impulse control;
- psychiatric history or personality disorder.

NAI is not necessarily inflicted by parent(s). It may be inflicted by baby-sitters, a cohabitee or transient partner, siblings or strangers.

Generally the perpetrator of NAI is well known to the victim

In dental aspects of NAI it is important that the dentist bears in mind that the injury may not have been inflicted by the parent(s). School-children have been known to carry out attacks leading to injury to the teeth and oral tissues. When presented with trauma that has apparently occurred at school, the dentist should note the time and circumstances of the injury and also who was involved. The authors have come across cases of sexual abuse by schoolchildren on a victim that presented as oral damage. This was a result of systematic abuse over a long period of time. Any case of dental trauma must always initially be considered as suspicious until the dentist is convinced otherwise.

There are various categories of abuse, of which physical trauma is only one. Sometimes several categories will occur in NAI to a child. Thus physical and sexual abuse may be associated with neglect. The dentist will in reality only be concerned with trauma and neglect, but all the categories are listed here for completeness:

- **Physical** – when a non-accidental act causes injury to the body of a child.
- **Neglect** – the negligent treatment or maltreatment of a child so that their health, welfare and safety are harmed.
- **Sexual** – covers a broad range of sexual acts perpetrated on children.
- **Emotional** – includes any behaviour which endangers the child's health, moral or emotional well-being.
- **Drugs** – which involves the administration of drugs or substances that are harmful and not intended for a child.

PHYSICAL ABUSE

Signs of physical abuse

The signs of physical abuse are many and varied. The dentist should be aware of bruises, burns, scalds and wounds to the face and head (Figure 14.1). However, it is quite possible for a dentist also to examine hands, arms and legs, particularly when clothing is easily displaced to reveal these parts of the body. Any suspicion of injury not commensurate with normal wear and tear, or rough and tumble, of children's activities should be investigated in detail.

Bruising

- Seen in 90% of abused children and usually there will be a number of bruises of different levels of healing.
- Normally rare in young immobile children.

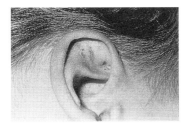

Figure 14.1 Photograph of bruising to an ear which could be seen by a dentist (courtesy Dr J. Wynn)

Table 14.1 Bruising of different ages

Age of bruise	Colour
0–48 hours	Red/purple – swollen tender
2–3 days	Purple/yellow
4–7 days	Yellow/brown
>7 days	Brown/fading

- Common over a bony prominence if a child has fallen, less common in softer areas of the body if bruises are sustained in normal childhood play.
- May have bruises of different ages, indicating more than one episode of abuse (Table 14.1).

Orofacial bruising may be seen on the scalp, forehead, cheeks, behind the ears, on an ear lobe or around the neck. These are all areas not commonly bruised from falling or knocking into objects during normal childhood activities.

Differential diagnosis of bruising is as follows:

- accidents;
- paint, ink;
- mongolian blue spot;
- bleeding disorder, such as idiopathic thrombocytopenic purpura, haemophilia, capillary haemangioma;
- rare conditions, such as leukaemia.

Dentists should also be aware that in some cultural practices, such as Chaio-Chaio (Vietnamese), objects (coins) are rubbed on the body to cure disease, producing superficial bruising.

Beating

The pattern of inflicted beating may be recognized as:

- multiple linear marks;
- buckle, belt marks;
- hand marks;
- marks by whips, chains, ropes;
- bizarre marks.

Knife wounds

There can be cuts and lacerations which may on occasion be inflicted on the face or forehead. These wounds may be bizarre in shape, such as stars or symbols, which are cut into a child's face. These have been know to have a ritual significance. In these circumstances explanations may be given, by parents or carers, that are peculiar and do not fit the pattern of injury. The authors were once asked to see a child, for damaged primary incisors, where there was an associated star-shaped cut on the forehead. The explanation given was that the child slipped and fell down stairs, hitting his head on the carved wooden newel post which caused the odd-shaped wound. Subsequent investigation revealed that a teenage baby-sitter had inflicted the wound with a Stanley knife. Dentists should therefore be aware that stories are readily made up to explain injuries in order to disguise NAI.

Burns

Interpretation of thermal injury may be difficult, especially if presentation is delayed. Burns are caused by dry heat, typically by cigarettes or cigars. However, other forms of heat have been used, as well as friction burns from ropes or chains.

Items to look out for include:

- cigarette burns – circular 0.5–1.0 cm;
- contact burn – shape conforms to object, such as hot radiators, irons, etc.;
- friction burns – superficial over body points, nose, shoulder, forehead.

Scalds

Scalds are caused by wet heat. They are often premeditated as a punishment to a young child, for instance where there are problems with toilet training. The dentist should watch out for:

- Accidental scalds, which have splash marks evident.
- Clear demarcated scalds, which imply dipping.

However, scalds are rarely seen on the face.

Bone injuries

Bone fractures are caused by trauma and may lead to loss of function in a limb. Skull fractures are often associated with head injury and retinal haemorrhages. Genuinely accidental fractures are usually simple skull fractures or transverse or greenstick fractures of the limbs. In contrast, multiple fractures in small children, which are rare without adequate explanation, such as a car accident, may be the result of NAI.

Intracranial injuries

These injuries will only rarely be seen by the general dental practitioner. There may, however, be a history of such injuries resulting in hospital admissions. A history of such injuries, together with the presentation of trauma to the teeth, should make a dentist suspicious and investigate further the aetiology of the presenting dental injury.

Scars to the skin around the hairline or upper face, easily looked at by a dentist, may be indicative of past injuries. In a young child these scars will appear white as they will not have had time to blend into the skin.

Sequelae and aspects of cranial injuries

- Injury to the brain is the commonest cause of death in child abuse.
- The majority of deaths occur in the first year of life.
- Uncommon after minor falls or even falls down stairs.
- Usually as a result of shaking and an impact.

Fractures of the facial bones

Whenever NAI is suspected and there is evidence of considerable trauma to the facial tissues and teeth, associated injuries to the bones of the face should be considered. In children, fractures of the mandibular condyles are uncommon. A sweeping blow to the lower jaw can give rise to unilateral or bilateral condylar fractures. Children who are pushed off furniture and fall on their face may also sustain such injuries.

Diagnosis is made by examination of the facial bones and assessment of movements of the mandible. Radiographs to show the condyles should be taken. An orthopantomogram (OPT) can be used for this purpose.

Facial stare

This is seen in victims of repeated abuse and is described as '*a vacant facial stare*' (Speight, 1989). The child in effect switches off from the events around him or her in an attempt not to attract further abuse. The child does not respond, or only very slowly, to questions by the dentist and appears to be divorced from the situation. It is characteristic of repeated abuse – physical, verbal or emotional.

Examination of the head and neck for NAI

As noted previously, a dentist who is suspicious of NAI should always examine those parts of a child's head and neck that are easily accessible. The scalp should be examined for torn hair, the ears for bruising, the eyes for retinal haemorrhage and the face and neck for old scars or bruising (Figure 14.2).

Orofacial injuries

Dentists will be most concerned by orofacial trauma in young children (Welbury and Murphy, 1998a). The injuries typically will present as damaged primary teeth. However, a torn frenum or bruising to the soft tissue of the mouth may also occur and should be noted with care in the light of a thorough history.

Violence is often directed at the mouth, as the child speaks or cries through it's mouth. A very common trauma occurs when a parent or abuser hits out at the child with the back of the hand or some sort of implement. In doing so, the teeth and lips are struck violently. If the

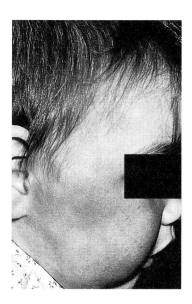

Figure 14.2 Photograph showing bruising to face – evidence of previous trauma (courtesy Dr J. Wynn)

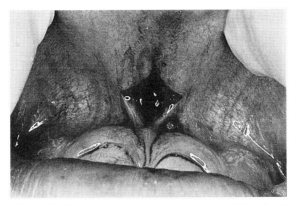

Figure 14.3 Photograph showing torn frenum in a child victim of NAI

motion is sweeping and upward, the maxillary frenum is torn at the same time as the lips and/or teeth are damaged. Radiographs of the teeth and facial bones may show signs of previous trauma.

These cases present as:

- Lips – bruising and laceration.
- Mucosa – torn frenum (Figure 14.3); also common in cases of forced feeding.
- Tongue – scarred or deviated; previous trauma.
- Teeth – discoloured and fractured, or knocked out.
- Occlusion – deranged occlusion.

DENTAL NEGLECT

Signs of neglect are:

- Child is underweight and malnourished.
- Pale muddy complexion.
- Poor hygiene – including oral hygiene.
- Inappropriately dressed for the weather conditions.
- Retarded physical or emotional development.
- Rampant caries.
- Untreated pain, infection or bleeding.
- Lack of continuity of care in the presence of identified dental pathology.

While it remains debatable as to whether severe dental disease in a young child is part of neglect, nevertheless a child with a dentition destroyed by extensive dental caries is unable to eat properly and will fail to thrive. Therefore, in the authors' opinion a severely carious primary dentition for which no attempt has been made to seek professional care by the parents or carers is a case of abuse. Dentitions decayed down to the gingival margin line (Figure 14.4) mean that a child is experiencing, or will have experienced, chronic pain.

Relevance to dentistry

In the survey by the NSPCC, some 50% of the abused children had suffered orofacial injuries. Therefore, the dentist may be the first person to see an abused child. While it is obvious that not every child who attends a dentist with orofacial trauma is a victim of NAI, a dentist should always be aware of the possibility.

Accordingly, the history that is taken for every trauma case (see Chapter 1) must be of sufficient detail that it records all previous instances of trauma. This situation also includes suspected cases of neglect.

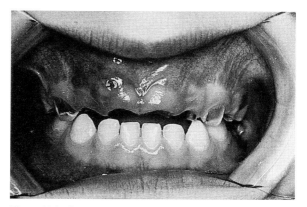

Figure 14.4 Photograph showing a badly broken down and neglected dentition of a pre-school child, who proved already to be under the care of social services because of general neglect

MANAGEMENT OF A CHILD PRESENTING WITH SUSPECTED NAI

The key points to remember about taking a history in suspected NAI are:

- Never accuse the parents of lying or being the perpetrators of NAI.
- Take the history carefully and in detail.
- Complete a trauma form.
- Check the history several times, but in different ways, to ensure consistency of aetiology.

The history should include:

- Detailed history of pain/injury.
- Detailed account of alleged accident, including records of the parents' explanation, when and where the alleged incident happened, what time, what exactly was the detailed sequence of events, who else witnessed the incident, etc?
- Medical history – check for any history of bleeding disorders and beware that some conditions, such as osteogenesis imperfecta, mimic NAI.
- Family and social history – record previous accidents.

A dentist should be wary of:

- Long, unexplained delay between accident and presentation for dental treatment.
- Explanation not consistent with injuries or a complete lack of explanation.
- Dental history changes and is inconsistent with the pattern of trauma.
- Parents touchy, irritable or evasive when asked questions.
- Parents giving inconsistent answers.

Examination

General observations should include:

- Facial expression, exposed skin.
- Appropriate clothing for time of the year; long sleeves may be hiding scars/bruises.
- Face and head – check scalp, eyes, face, neck, ears and throat for bruising, bites, burns, scars, etc.
- Oral – lips, mucosa, teeth, evidence of intra-oral scarring, bruising.
- Gait on entering surgery – limping or hesitant.

Records

Detailed documentation at the time of the dental examination is vital, even if the dentist is hard-pressed in a busy clinic. As with all cases of trauma, the use of the trauma form is highly recommended, as we have repeated many times throughout this textbook.

The witnesses to the completion of the history and dental records should be noted. In most cases this will be the dental nurse. It is useful for the dental nurse to ask similar questions as the dentist concerning the history, when the dentist has left the surgery, to perhaps see another patient or process a radiograph, etc.

If two parents or carers are present in a case of suspected NAI, one can be taken elsewhere on an excuse for completing a form, etc., while the other is re-questioned on the history. By these means a history can be cross-checked for consistency.

The following details should be recorded

- Names and addresses of all people accompanying the child.
- Time of arrival.
- Illustrations of the size, position and type of injuries.
- Photographic documentation is beneficial in this respect, although it is recognized that not all dentists have a suitable camera.

Suspicions may also be aroused by a history that does not make sense. In a case recently seen by the authors, for example, a story was told of how a child fell off a kitchen table onto their father's bicycle. Is it usual for a bicycle to be in a kitchen? What was the child doing on the top of a kitchen table? The story seemed unlikely and further investigation revealed a family registered with social services as being under surveillance for possible NAI.

Management and official reporting of NAI

This is the crucial issue for dentists. What should they do about reporting cases of suspected NAI? Many dentists will be hesitant to get involved and feel that they might be making a wrong diagnosis. They will be concerned about any possible legal repercussions that might backfire on them. Adverse publicity might well affect their public image. Fortunately there are now systems in place whereby a dentist can report such cases without the suspected abusing parents or carers being aware of the report. An excellent outline of procedures has been published by Welbury and Murphy (1998b) and this proforma for dealing with suspected NAI is shown at the end of this chapter.

Local guidelines can usually be obtained from Social Services or at departments of paediatrics at local hospitals. Other sources of contact and information include:

- Consultants in Paediatric Dentistry.
- Community Paediatricians.
- Senior Dental Officers (SDOs) in Paediatric Dentistry.
- District Dental Officer in the Community Dental Services.
- Social Services.

Consultants in Paediatric Dentistry and SDOs in Paediatric Dentistry will be well versed in the reporting procedures because of the nature of their training and specialization.

The **sequence of events** when a suspected case of NAI is encountered is as follows:

- Take **history**, using trauma form.
- Complete **dental examination**.
- Take any necessary **radiographs and photographs**.
- Commence **emergency treatment** of any trauma.
- **Re-check history** for consistency.
- Ensure **safety of the child** if abuse is suspected; provide help for the parents, which usually involves a referral.
- **Call** Social Services or the Community Paediatrician and ask if there is any record of the child/family being known or any previous history of trauma.
- Arrange for a **recall appointment**, preferably in 1 week, as a follow-up.

Referral

If the injuries are severe and the child requires specialized treatment or hospitalization, the child should be referred to the local Accident and Emergency Department (it is a good idea to telephone and advise the department of the child's imminent arrival). As noted in the bullet points above, find out if patient is known to Social Services; either telephone Social Services, or the community paediatric department in the local hospital and ask to speak to the designated consultant who deals with cases of child abuse. If the referral is made to the Social Services department this will need to be confirmed in writing. The child's medical practitioner should also be informed. Advice can also be sought from the nearest consultant or senior dental officer in paediatric dentistry who will be able to advise on procedures or take over the case on behalf of the general dental practitioner.

If there is a history or record of the child and family, a report should be written and kept on file. It is useful for a copy of the report to be sent in strict confidence to the appropriate department of community paediatrics. In many countries, such as the USA, a dental surgeon is immune to litigation over unsubstantiated diagnosis of NAI, but this is not so in all countries. The dentist should therefore in all instances work through the appropriate authorities such as Community Paediatrics or Social Services.

Under no circumstances should the dentist accuse the parents/ carers of NAI or intimate to them in any way his or her suspicions

Always work through and with the appropriate authorities. On the other hand, the **worst thing that can be done for a child with NAI is nothing**. General dental practitioners should not feel guilty about referring children with suspected NAI. They are not accusing either parent; they are simply asking for a second opinion on an important diagnosis.

Follow-up

At a subsequent appointment, the treatment is continued. If, however, the child fails to attend this, it is important and should be noted. If contact has been made with Community Paediatric or Social Services, they should be notified of the failure to attend.

SUMMARY

General dental practitioners should always be aware that children presenting with dental trauma might be a victim of NAI. Practitioners should be familar with warning signs of NAI, complete accurate and detailed records and notify the relevant authorities, without jeopardizing the well-being of the child. Dental trauma due to NAI should be dealt with speedily.

REFERENCES AND FURTHER READING

Becker, D.B., Needlemann, H.L. and Kotelchuck, M. (1978) Child abuse and dentistry: oro-facial trauma and its recognition by dentists. *Journal of the American Dental Association*, **97**, 24–28

Hobbs, C.J. and Wynn, J.M. (1996) Head and eye injuries. In *Physical Signs of Child Abuse. A Colour Atlas.* W.B. Saunders, London

Meadow, R. (1989) *The ABC of Child Abuse.* British Medical Journal Publications, London

Murphy, J.M. and Welbury, R.R. (1998) The dental practitioner's role in protecting children from abuse. 1. The Child Protection System. *British Dental Journal*, **184**, 7–10

Speight, N. (1989) Non-accidental injury. In *ABC of Child Abuse* (edited by R. Meadow). British Medical Publications, London

Welbury, R.R. and Murphy, J.M. (1998a) The dental practitioner's role in protecting children from abuse. 2. The oro-facial signs of abuse. *British Dental Journal*, **184**, 61–65

Welbury, R.R. and Murphy, J.M. (1998b) The dental practitioner's role in protecting children from abuse. 3. Reporting and subsequent management of abuse. *British Dental Journal*, **184**, 115–119

(See over for **Guidelines for Dental Practitioners on Child Protection**)

GUIDELINES FOR DENTAL PRACTITIONERS ON CHILD PROTECTION

These guidelines are reproduced as a quick reference for dentists. They are designed so that if a dentist is suspicious that NAI may have occurred in a child presenting with dental trauma, the procedures for reporting can be quickly cross-checked. It is suggested that these guidelines could be copied and included as part of the operating procedures of the dental practice.

What to do if there are concerns giving rise to suspicions of child abuse

---

It is vital that all concerned with infants and young children should be alert for the signs of child abuse. However, it should also be remembered that older children are not immune. Children are also subject to other forms of abuse besides physical which include sexual and emotional abuse. Warning signs of these kinds of abuse may not come from a physical injury and will require:

- Observations of the nature of the relationship between parent and child.
- The child's reaction to other people.
- The child's reaction to dental and medical examinations.
- The general demeanour of the child.
- Any comments made by the child and/or parent or carer that give concern about the child's upbringing or lifestyle.

Some of the earliest signs of physical ill-treatment of children are to be found in facial bruising and damage to and around the mouth. It is essential that general dental practitioners play a responsible role in any arrangements made to record potential danger to children arising from ill-treatment by parent or anybody having care of children. Where the child is found with a physical injury, no matter how minor, the dentist should ask the following questions:

- Could the injury have been caused accidentally? If so, how?
- If an explanation for an injury is given, does the injury fit in with the facts?
- If there has been a delay in seeking dental care, on the part of the parents/carers, are there good reasons for this?
- If the explanation of cause is consistent with the injury, is this cause itself within normal acceptable limits of behaviour?

Who do general dental practitioners consult for suspected NAI?

For all cases where there is suspicion of possible abuse, dentists should seek the advice of:

- Consultant in paediatric dentistry – at nearest hospital.
- Consultant in community paediatrics – at nearest hospital.
- Consultant in dental public health (or their authorized deputies).

Dentists working in the Community Dental Service should contact their nearest Senior Dental Officer in paediatric dentistry or dental services manager.

What steps should be taken?

In those cases where suspicions are aroused, the following steps will need to be taken according to the location of the dental examination:

- In the case of a child examined or treated in a pre-school or play group, nursery school or school, the head teacher or play group leader should be informed.
- In the case of a child being examined in any other location, such as a clinic or dental surgery (office), the child's general medical practitioner or community paediatrician (cross-referenced to the relevant sections of these guidelines) should be told, in order to arrange for a medical examination.

The reasons for suspicions should be given.

When and how should this information be given?

Direct contact should be made in person or by telephone with the community paediatrician or general medical practitioner in the case of children treated within clinics or a dental surgery (office). The head teacher should also be contacted directly or by telephone in cases where children have been treated or examined in schools. These people should be contacted immediately.

What are the requirements for record keeping?

All records of the visits, dental and medical history, and discussions, should be recorded in full. The trauma form should be used. In some circumstances it may be necessary to provide diagrams or even photographs. The records should be completed immediately.

Who makes the decision on future action?

The head teacher/play group leader is responsible for further action in the case of children examined in pre-schools, play groups, nursery schools or schools.

For those children who have been treated in any other location, such as a clinic or dental surgery (office), the community paediatrician or general medical practitioner should be responsible for further action. However, in extreme conditions where these cannot be contacted and immediate action is called for, the dentist should contact a local hospital's paediatrics department and arrange for the child to be seen. The child's general medical practitioner should be informed of this action.

What action occurs from this point?

Following a referral to either a head teacher/play group leader or general medical practitioner, a *referral of concern* will be made to social services, if considered appropriate.

What is the dentist's responsibility for follow-up?

For those children who have been treated within a clinic or dental surgery (office), the community paediatrician or general medical practitioner should be contacted within 24 hours to check that the child has been seen.

It may be necessary to refer to the records in any subsequent case conference or court proceedings, so it is vitally important that a full record is made at the time of the dental examination. All parts of the **trauma form** should therefore be completed. Notes should be made on who has been contacted and what was discussed.

After Welbury and Murphy (1998b), reproduced by permission of the *British Dental Journal*.

Index